Remembering Mark

Dancing in the Sky

Colleen Nuncio

outskirts
press

Acknowledgments

This book is dedicated to my daughter, **Lynn Ostrander Harris Dunn,** who was by my side throughout Mark's journey, and to my son, **Kevin Ostrander**, who was truly his brother's keeper and rescued Mark during many critical times in his life.

Thanks to **Mark's family,** who supported him from the beginning to the end of his eventful journey.

Thanks to Mark's best friend, **Mark (Roz) Rosdail**, who remained a true friend throughout good times and bad.

Thanks to **Mindy (Malinda) Rosdail-Johnson,** who was an integral part of Mark's life and with whom he shared his innermost thoughts and feelings.

Thanks to my compassionate boss, **Tom Cordner**, whose understanding made it possible for me to visit Mark every day on my lunch break from work.

Thanks to my mentor, **Brandi Cooper,** for encouraging me to write Mark's story and put it before the public.

Thanks to my editor, **Diane Baumer**, a true professional who made the final edits to this book and made it easy to read and understand.

Special thanks to my husband, **Martin,** for his patience and support while I spent many hours poring over Mark's biography.

Table of Contents

Preface

MENTAL ILLNESS IS a biological disorder that strikes one out of every four families. It can be devastating, and many times tears families apart. Research of diseases of the brain has been far behind that of other biological illnesses. It is only recently that help has begun to surface for mental illnesses such as bipolar disorder (manic depression), clinical depression, and Haslam-Pinnell Syndrome (schizophrenia).

From 1989 through 1994, I was secretary of the Dallas Alliance for the Mentally Ill (at the time known as TEXAMI). It is now an affiliate of the National Alliance on Mental Illness (NAMI). NAMI is a grassroots, self-help support and advocacy organization of families and friends of people with serious mental illnesses. Its mission is to eradicate mental illness and to improve the quality of life for those who suffer from no-fault brain diseases. NAMI is a non-profit, 501(c)(3) corporation, and funds raised are used to benefit seriously mentally ill people and their families.

In June of 1991, when I was living in Dallas, Texas, my son, Mark, who had been battling bipolar disorder for nearly ten years, became unstable and entered into a confrontation with a SWAT team in Iowa. Mark was violently throwing things around his second-floor apartment, down the stairs, and out the windows. When local law enforcement officers arrived, he came downstairs and threatened them with clubs. He then ran back upstairs and held the officers at bay by flinging objects down the narrow stairwell. That is when the decision was made to call in the state tactical team. The episode was reported in several Iowa newspapers, and the stigma associated with mental illness helped to fuel the public's interest. At that time, of all 50 states, Iowa was the only state with a county-based funding system for mental illness. Other states that received federal tax dollars also received matching funds from the federal government, making possible crisis intervention, vocational rehabilitation, and social programs. These programs were desperately needed in Iowa. Thanks to current research and public education, the stigma that has been associated with mental illness is gradually being removed. Still, progress is painfully slow and inadequate.

Introduction

MARK BEGAN WRITING his story while in a nursing home on September 27, 2015. Sadly, two years later, he succumbed to the ravages of mental illness and passed away, leaving an unfinished end to his writings. This collaboration between mother and son is a collection of his memories and the random thoughts he penned throughout the course of his 56 years on earth.

On December 27th, 1994, I decided that I no longer wanted to live with my bipolar disorder. Diagnosed when I was 21, I had endured it for 13 years when I decided to end my life. Since that time, I have been in no less than 40 hospitals, rehab facilities, and nursing homes due to injuries sustained from an unsuccessful suicide attempt. After I jumped from a balcony, I ended up with a traumatic brain injury and broken left leg. I received brain surgery, and a plate and screws were placed in my left leg.

My experiences in nursing homes left a great deal to be desired.

This was the beginning of what was to have been Mark's message to his friends and relatives, letting them know that he had chosen not to live. His way of saying good-bye.

This book is a tribute to my son, Mark, a talented, gifted, intelligent, and courageous young man whose life was destroyed by mental illness. It describes what people with mental illness and their families go through, their suicide attempts, and the exasperating, too often unfulfilled search for proper treatment. You will read what he was forced to deal with in the nursing homes—the usual "last resort" for many who need a place to live.

These chapters are arranged chronologically so you can follow Mark's chaotic journey as he struggled to pull his life together, fulfill his dreams, and meet his own high expectations as he attempted to lend a semblance of order and stability to his life. Mark had the support of his entire family and friends while going through the hell he was living. The National Alliance on Mental Illness (NAMI) was a continued source of strength and guidance as I sought help for Mark.

May you benefit from Mark's experiences by learning to recognize when persons with mental illness need help and knowing you are not alone if you find yourself or your friends and family in similar circumstances.

CHAPTER 1

Early Childhood
through Junior College
1962–1981

MARK'S CHILDHOOD SEEMED normal. I did not detect any unusual behaviors that would have alerted me to him having any medical or psychiatric disorders. Mark's biological father and I were divorced in 1962 when Mark was two years of age, and he was adopted by my second husband, Denny Ostrander. At times he seemed extremely sensitive and cried easily—once when he missed a music competition and another time when Denny and I informed him and his siblings that we were getting a divorce. At the time, those emotions seemed reasonable to me, since these were significant events in Mark's life.

Mark's academic abilities revealed themselves through good grades from kindergarten through high school, where he placed on the Honor Roll and then throughout college, where he was on the Dean's List and earned his Associate Degree in Science.

His talent for music became apparent by age ten when he received an "Excellent" rating in the drum competition at the grade school music festival. Later in high school, he played drums in the Osage Iowa Drum & Bugle Corps. He also lettered in track, wrestling, and football in both junior and senior high school. An outstanding wrestler, Mark wrestled on the senior varsity team while he was in junior high school. So handsome with his blond hair, blue eyes, toned body, and infectious smile, he represented his class as Homecoming King. He had an exuberant zest for life–with a positive attitude that inspired others.

When I was 18, my dance partner and I won a contest in northeast Iowa for a trip to Hollywood. We danced on the Dance Fever TV show. I was about the best dancer at the Runway Disco. Because my Mom taught me all the fancy moves. And the women there just loved being shown off. My sister, Lynn, and I once won the talent show in Clear Lake, Iowa. When I attended North Iowa Area Community College in Mason City, I met my best friend Mark Rosdail. My girlfriend just happens to be his sister. I went to two colleges in Iowa. I wanted to become a dentist, but my bipolar illness got in the way.

First Breakdown and Hospitalizations

1981–1984

AFTER BEGINNING HIS junior year in college, Mark took a break from school and spent the summer in Maine with his biological father and family (whom he had never met). The visit went exceptionally well, and Mark was welcomed into the lives of his biological father, stepmother, half-sisters, aunts, and uncles. Years later, he remained in touch with them through email and by telephone. Weeks after visiting his family, he moved to Atlantic City, NJ, where he worked as a sales representative on The Boardwalk.

While in New Jersey, Mark called me and seemed extremely upset that his sister, Lynn, and adoptive father, Denny, could not visit him as they had planned. When I visited him later that summer, he was very active in his job and spent very little time with me, but seemed happy and was thoroughly engrossed in his work.

In September, even though Mark had not planned to go to college in the fall, I was surprised when he called and informed me that he was back in school at the University of Iowa. In subsequent calls to me, Mark tearfully expressed how very lonely he was. His thoughts raced, and he said that he wished he hadn't taken street drugs (Mescaline) on his drive home from Atlantic City.

A month later, Mark called me from school and was crying; he seemed terrified. Mark's brother Kevin, his friend, and I drove to Iowa City to visit him. When we arrived at his fraternity house, we noticed marijuana cigarettes lying on the table. At first, we thought Mark was under the influence of drugs.

I used to love illegal drugs. Pot was my first use–at NIACC, the community college that I attended. I usually smoked Marlboro cigarettes. I was introduced to cocaine at the Runway Disco, where I worked. I've never tried heroin, but it's a good thing because I understand it is very addictive.

During our conversation, Mark wasn't making a lot of sense, with rapid, disjointed, and fleeting thoughts. One moment he would appear in control; the next, he would be crying and confused. We realized that Mark was not himself and convinced him to take a break from school and come home for a while.

As the four of us were driving home–Kevin and his friend in the front seat, Mark and I in the back–Mark had episodes of weeping. When I asked him why he was crying, he replied, "I'm afraid."

"Why are you afraid?"

"I don't know."

We would come to understand that Mark, now at age 21, had begun an uphill battle with mental illness, which would eventually force him to withdraw from his junior year in college.

Over the next few days, Mark acted out of character; he was belligerent and paranoid. After taking my car without permission, he spent the night of November 2nd with his brother in Mason City, Iowa. In the middle of the night, Mark told Kevin, "I can't close my eyes." Kevin suggested that Mark go to the hospital emergency room for a check-up. Mark agreed and was admitted to the St. Joseph Mercy Hospital from November 3-12. He received a diagnosis of schizoaffective disorder during his stay, but as Mark spent time in different hospitals, his diagnoses changed. Eventually, he was diagnosed with bipolar disorder.

Mark was discharged from the hospital on November 12th but re-entered the hospital on December 3rd when he became unstable. He was released again on December 14th. Side effects from medication were horrendous: rapid pulse, high blood pressure, headaches, leg tremors, blurred vision, and restlessness. From 11/11/81-1/3/82, Mark was given Haldol, Cogentin, Sodium Amytal, Prolixin, Elavil, and Valium.

On January 3, 1982, I had Mark referred to Mayo Clinic in Rochester, Minnesota, for a complete medical and neurological examination. While there, all medication was discontinued. Mark was tearful and depressed most of the time. Although the doctors preferred that Mark remain in the hospital for more observation, he was discharged after two weeks because he felt he wasn't making any progress. His leg tremors, blurred vision, and tearfulness were subsiding. His blood pressure and pulse rate improved.

Mark started to see a psychologist in Mason City, Iowa, once a week. He had gained 50 pounds—a side effect of the medication. Most of the time, he withdrew from any contact with friends; therefore, he had no social life. He continued to progress though, and began to jog and exercise.

In June, Mark and I moved from Osage, Iowa, to Dallas, Texas. He continued to improve and acquired a job with Tejas Architectural Products, becoming more outgoing and making friends.

By fall, Mark had lost 50 pounds with the aid of over-the-counter diet drugs (Dexatrim) and very little food. He became progressively more active and started having trouble sleeping, as well as becoming very unpredictable. I suspected he was using street drugs with his friends.

On November 14th, Mark moved out of the apartment that we shared with my sister. Two days later, he returned and called his friend. He was crying and speaking irrationally, and on November 21st, he moved back into our apartment. The next day he quit his job and began driving to Iowa. He only made it as far as Topeka, Kansas. On November 23rd, the police picked him up at a truck stop where he had been bothering people for several hours. Under an order of protective custody, he was admitted to Topeka State Hospital. Two days later, Mark was with me.

Less than a week later, on November 27th, Mark became verbally abusive and demonstrated no sense of responsibility. The next day he went to his friend's apartment and began to fight with him; that resulted in his being jailed for disorderly conduct, resisting arrest, and failure to show identification.

On the 29th, I went to the mental illness (M.I.) department to get an M.I. warrant filed so Mark could go directly to Parkland Hospital when he was released from jail. A social worker suggested I get Mark out of jail on the condition that Mark would seek counseling on his own the following day.

Mark was released from jail on December 3rd. The "resisting arrest" charge was reduced to "class 3 assault." On December 4th, Mark and I drove to Terrell State Hospital in Terrell, Texas. Mark was verbally abusive most of the way. When we arrived at the hospital gate, Mark began to cry, and he asked me to drive. When we met with a doctor, Mark assumed that the visit was for an evaluation. When we explained to him that he would have to admit himself for the formal evaluation, he refused.

I told Mark that I was leaving to drive back to Dallas. Before I left, I went back into the hospital to make a phone call and discovered that Mark was using the telephone to call a cab, so I left. Mark followed me to the car and threatened to fight me for the keys. Again, I went into the hospital and asked the security officer to accompany me to my car. Mark took his belongings from the car, and sadness overwhelmed me as I drove away. I felt as though I was abandoning my son.

At 2:30 a.m., Mark called and threatened to harm me. My sister and I were frightened, so we spent the rest of the night away from our apartment; I stayed with my niece, and Joan stayed with her friend. At 6:00 a.m., Mark knocked on the door where Joan had spent the night and told her that he had damaged a clock, a telephone, and a lamp, which we later found was untrue. He also told her that I should stay out of his way. I called the police and tried to get an M.I. warrant but was unable to since Mark's charges had been reduced. I went to the M.I. department and signed for a warrant again, but learned that Mark was back in jail, so the warrant was invalid. I was advised to leave Mark in jail and get a peace bond or restraining order so he could not bother us when he was released. How frustrating! Mark needed to be hospitalized–not thrown in jail!

I met with the judge to inquire about a peace bond. He said that a peace bond was not the answer and referred me to a different judge. On December 9th, the second judge called me and agreed to sign an M.I. warrant. The next day I signed the warrant, which was good for two weeks, and took it to the sheriff's department; Mark was taken from jail directly to Parkland Hospital Emergency Room, and his evaluation was scheduled to take two to three days. A court date was set in case Mark refused treatment or if doctors decided he needed it. At last! Mark would be getting the help he desperately needed!

On December 11th, Mark was admitted to Hillside Mental Diagnostic Center. Five days later, he was admitted to Terrell State Hospital. When the 90-day commitment expired on March 16, 1983, Mark voluntarily extended his stay until August. He was finally discharged on August 31, 1983, and moved to Storm Lake, Iowa, where he began employment at Iowa Beef Producers (I.B.P.)

For the next two years, Mark remained stable and functioned well in his job, where he operated robotic equipment and supervised product movement between departments. He won management recognition for superior effort involving a 12-man crew.

I ran the box room when I worked there. It was full of computers that printed on the side of each box what it contained and what it weighed. And we really scrambled our butts off when things went wrong! All the big wigs tried their best to help. Because that was a lot of meat to be dealing with.

A relationship developed between Mark and his co-worker, and they lived together with her 3-year old son through the fall of 1985.

I met her while we were working at I.B.P. The relationship ended when I broke up with her because her ex came around and wanted to be her son's father. But we sure had a lot of fun while we were together.

CHAPTER 3

Four Years of Roller Coaster Existence

1985–1989

IN THE FALL of 1985, Mark re-enrolled in The University of Iowa and changed his major from pre-dentistry to electrical engineering. By the beginning of the second semester, he could not focus on his studies and had to withdraw from college. He moved to Floyd, Iowa, and lived with his grandparents. As they worked together, restoring Mark's truck, he and his grandfather developed a deep bond. The following year Mark moved to Mason City, Iowa, and began employment at The Pheasant Run Supper Club. Under his doctor's supervision, he began to reduce his Lithium and appeared to be functioning well on 600 mg/day.

By March 1987, Mark became involved in the Jehovah's Witness religion. He discontinued Lithium and gave two weeks' notice that he was quitting his job. After donating some of his belongings to his friends, he left other possessions in his apartment and began walking in a southerly direction.

On March 29th, police contacted Mark's brother, Kevin, in Osage, IA, and informed him of Mark's irrational behavior. The next day, with snow on the ground from a severe snowstorm that had occurred two days prior, Mark was discovered wandering in the streets with no coat and no shoes. Kevin was there to help take care of Mark's affairs when, on April 2, 1987, Mark was hospitalized for the seventh time due to his mental illness. He was admitted to Cherokee Mental Health Institute, where he was treated for two months.

On June 5th Mark was released into my custody and moved to Texas to live with my husband, Martin, and me.

Mark was able to manage his daily medications - 2100mg Lithium Carbonate/day (mood stabilizer); 40mg Navane/day (antipsychotic); 2mg Cogentin/day (anti-tremor to decrease hand tremors and muscle stiffness–side effects of antipsychotic meds) – but they made him very drowsy, and he needed to sleep a lot. Unable to drive, his physical movements were very stiff and mechanical, he had slight hand tremors, and reacted slowly to external stimuli. Mark found it very difficult to become motivated to do anything, remaining extremely depressed, with feelings of worthlessness.

The first appointment with his social worker and doctor at Dallas Mental Health Clinic on Routh Street was on June 23rd. His social worker made arrangements to enroll him in an adult day treatment program, which began August 11th.

Unable to work, Mark had to apply for financial aid to survive. On August 15th, Mark and I had a hearing with an administrative law judge to request financial assistance. From late August until late December, Mark and I had also met several times with representatives of the Social Security Office and Texas Rehabilitation Commission (TRC). In October, Social Security denied Mark benefits; he reapplied in December.

By August 23rd, Mark was totally unhappy with the treatment center and said he didn't want to go on with his life. His doctor had been gradually reducing his medication, and by September 22nd, the Navane had been discontinued. He continued to attend the adult treatment center until November 5th. In late December, Mark was accepted by TRC to enroll in Control Data Institute (CDI) for Computer Technology Training from January through September 1988.

Although school hours were from 7:30 a.m. until 12:30 p.m., Mark stayed nearly all day so he could stay on schedule and meet the deadline for his tests. He tried very hard to maintain a high grade point average. He got excellent grades on his tests, even though he had difficulty staying awake in class. Because Mark thought his medication was making him drowsy, his doctor reduced the dosage, which seemed to help. He also continued to complain of daily headaches and told the doctor, but was unable to get any relief from them.

With regular exercise (jogging, playing tennis, and swimming), Mark lost the weight that he had gained within the previous year. He took an interest in his personal appearance and looked great.

In April, Mark acquired part-time employment at MicroAge Computer Stores, Inc. as a computer technician while attending school in the morning. Initially concerned that his grades may suffer, he needn't have worried, as he maintained high grades, and he had excellent attendance. His job ended in July when Mark was laid off due to reduced company sales.

Mark was employed by Tigon in Far North Dallas on September 1, 1988. He was excited about his new job and was able to postpone school until he became oriented in his new position. His employer suggested that Mark work nights and finish school during the day since he was nearly finished.

On the weekend of September 10th, Mark went to Parkland Emergency to find relief from his persistent daily headaches to no avail. That same weekend he went to Robert H. Dedman (RHD) Hospital ER but found no relief. My personal physician performed several medical tests and prescribed Elavil. Mark believed that the headaches were a side effect of Lithium. He became increasingly irritable and showed a great deal of animosity toward me. I suspected he had not been taking his Lithium. He got upset and moved out. Until he was able to move into an apartment, he stayed with his sister, Lynn, in Lewisville, Texas.

Then…he quit his job.

On September 30th Mark called me at work and asked for a ride to school. During my lunch break, I picked him up at his apartment and proceeded to drive south on I-35. He became verbally abusive toward me in the car, was critical of everything I said, and became upset, accusing me of ignoring him and not talking to him when I nodded my head to acknowledge his questions and comments. Suddenly, he insisted that I stop the car and let him out–which I did.

At 7:00 p.m., I telephoned CDI to see if Mark had attended school that day. An instructor told me that Mark was at school from approximately 3:30 p.m. until 5:30 p.m. He also said that he was concerned about Mark, because he wasn't acting like himself; he seemed agitated and upset. I told him that I, too, was worried and was trying to locate him.

On that day, I received notice from the Department of Health and Human Services, Office of Hearings and Appeals, of a favorable decision from the administrative law judge granting Mark financial assistance. This came in a very timely manner, because it appeared that Mark was becoming unstable.

On October 1st, Mark called his sister Lynn and asked her to drive him to the Salvation Army. He told her that she must be at his apartment by 7:30 a.m., or he would not be there. When Lynn arrived, she said she barely knew Mark—he even appeared to be walking differently. He got in the car, and she proceeded to drive him to the Salvation Army. When she asked him why he was going to the Salvation Army, he replied that he needed a place to sleep and a hot meal. She complied with all of Mark's requests, because she felt afraid of him.

I called the Salvation Army, and a staff member verified that Mark was there. I told him of Mark's circumstances. The following day, I spoke with two counselors there; both men attempted to communicate with Mark. Two days later, I talked to Mark's social worker from Routh Street Clinic. She called a counselor from the Salvation Army, who personally escorted Mark to the Clinic to meet with her. She convinced Mark to take his medication, and it was agreed that Mark would stay at the Salvation Army while he attended school to take his final exam. The counselor informed me that Mark needed clothes to wear to school, so I took several changes of clothing to him. The next day, I was told that he tried to donate his clothing to the Salvation Army.

On October 8, 1988, Mark left the Salvation Army. He called Lynn and asked her to pick him up at the Holiday Inn at Mockingbird Lane and I-35. Lynn called me, and I immediately called the Salvation Army. I was informed that Mark had said that he was going out for a walk. Knowing that Mark was in a vulnerable position and may be in danger, I called the judge at Lew Sterett Jail, who issued a mental illness warrant for Mark. Because we didn't know Mark's whereabouts, I called the police and reported him missing. At approximately 2:30 a.m., police officers picked him up near Love Field Airport. He was walking in the middle of the street and was not wearing shoes. Mark asked them to call me and have me come and get him, but I told the officer that an M.I. warrant had been issued for Mark, so they drove him to Parkland Emergency.

The doctor at Parkland Hospital told my husband and me that Mark would be admitted to Mental Diagnostic Center (MDC) if he was not cooperative. The next day Mark was moved to MDC. His counselor reported Mark's progress to me each day. Mark did not contest the decision to go to Hillside, so he was admitted on October 14th for further evaluation. Two weeks later, he moved back into the Salvation Army while waiting for his Social Security check so he could move into Mae Smith's transitional house in Garland, TX. Side effects from his medication were noticeable–he was very restless and continually moved his legs. He also returned to Control Data Institute and took his final exams, which he passed with a GPA of 96.1.

On November 9th, while Mark was visiting us, he had a confrontation with Martin, and we told him he had to leave. Two days later Mark wrote us this letter:

Dear Nuncios,

I can't begin to know where to start. So I'll just say I'm homesick for both of you.

The reason I got into it with you, Martin, is because I was taking all my frustrations out on you. It really hurts me to think I'm not wanted somewhere.

I'm really scared to be on my own. It's really lonely sometimes. And I miss your 100 years of combined wisdom compared to my 28.

Whatever happens, know that you both have my deep respect and love. Mark

Mark received his Computer Technology Degree on November 22nd and moved to Mae Smith's transitional house in Garland on the 1st of December. On the 10th, Mark's sister Lynn, nephew Zach, and I attended Mark's graduation ceremony at Control Data Institute. He was stable, and it was a happy time.

On January 6, 1989, Mark began working at Protech Service Center in Richardson, TX. He was functioning well. His job was going great, and he continued attending computer seminars to further his computer technician career. He purchased a personal computer, which enabled him to develop expertise in all facets of his career, bought a car, and moved into his own apartment.

Romance entered his life once again. He and his girlfriend were very happy, and on Mark's birthday, April 29th, they invited Lynn's family and Martin and me to dinner at their apartment. These were happy times.

Then, danger signals reared their ugly heads. Mark's medication made him drowsy, so his new doctor tried another medication. On June 15th, he received bad news from Iowa: his grandfather had major cancer surgery, and Mark became quite concerned about him. By August, Mark became increasingly rude to me; it was nearly impossible to carry on a conversation with him. He would find fault with grammatical errors and would detect–and point out–all statements that seemed to him to be contradictory. And he found it hard to tolerate other people's ideas if they did not coincide with his own.

Mark's employer informed me that Mark had quit his job with Protech without notice, stating family problems and internal strife as his reasons for leaving. He left mid-morning on August 28th. Kevin, Mark's brother, called me from Iowa on August 30th and told me that Mark was in Iowa. He had stopped at Kevin's, and Mark tried to start a fight with him.

I telephoned the clinic to see if Mark had medication and was informed he had received a six-week supply of Lithium in July that should have lasted him until September. This time, it was my turn to terminate Mark's apartment lease, sell his furniture, and salvage what I could from his abrupt departure. It was another major setback as instability set in once again. It was also the end of another romantic relationship.

A reunion of family and friends was scheduled at Mark's grandparents' home on Labor Day weekend. Many family members were concerned that Mark may disrupt the event, but he assured us that he would not create a scene. During the reunion, Mark was at times hospitable and, at times, not. Mostly, he remained distant during the 3-day reunion. When I left, instead of his usual hug and goodbye kiss on the cheek, he shook my hand and seemed angry with me.

During the following weeks, Mark interviewed for several jobs and planned to begin a new one on Monday, October 2nd. Saturday night, September 30th, Mark's new girlfriend contacted me to tell me that

Mark was picked up by the police after complaints by several people that he was acting strangely. He was taken to the emergency room at Floyd County Memorial Hospital, and the doctor who examined him informed him that if he took his medication (Lithium), he could go home. An appointment was made for the following Tuesday for a follow-up visit. The ER nurse, an acquaintance of mine, said she had seen Mark at church services several days earlier.

Mark began his new job on Monday but was unable to follow instructions or function rationally. He was asked to leave mid-morning.

Tuesday, Mark's grandparents, Doris and Ralph Brown, tried to telephone Mark at his apartment in Charles City, Iowa, but could not reach him. They knew he had a doctor's appointment at 9:00 a.m., so drove to his residence and offered to take him. Mark declined the offer and would not invite them in even though they asked.

Wednesday, October 4th, Mark arrived at his grandparents' home in Floyd with all of his belongings (except the ones he had discarded) loaded into his car. He was ravenously hungry, so his grandmother prepared lunch for him. She said he ate as though he hadn't eaten for days. He told them he hadn't slept.

After becoming aggressive toward a neighbor, the police were notified, and Mark was taken to the Mental Health Institute (MHI) in Independence, Iowa. I telephoned MHI and gave the staff a summary of Mark's medical history, medication he was taking, and his doctor and case manager's contact information. The next day, October 5th, he was admitted.

The nurse told me that Mark had been in restraints most of the time since admission. He had been given Thorazine at 2:30, 7:00, and 11:00 a.m. I asked why Mark was not on Lithium; she didn't know and told me to ask the doctor. The doctor on call suggested several possible reasons and promised to confer with Mark's assigned doctor. The next day Mark was slightly improved; he was still in wrist-to-wrist restraints but was walking around. They also started him back on Lithium.

Mark's doctor and social worker kept me informed of Mark's progress. By November 15th, he was transferred to an open less-restrictive ward, got a work assignment, and was progressing well. Mark's social worker applied for his acceptance into North Iowa Transition Center in Mason City, Iowa, for supervised apartment living.

In the fall of 1989, Mark wrote me this letter:

Dear Mom,

You've been my truest friend for eight years—ever since all this crap started.

I'm going to let you in on a little secret. The reason I get so disgusted on the phone is because you remind me of things (stupid things) I've done, and I get real <u>disappointed in myself</u>.

You see, I've always wanted a family like "The Waltons."[1] Also, things aren't in perfect order. And you know how I have to have everything just right; I'm a perfectionist.

If you had asked me at age 21 what things would be like when I was 30, I would have said I'd be on top of the world. But here I am flat on my ass, not such a big shot anymore.

So I can't think of much else to say. I need to apologize, but I don't have the energy.

Thanks for doing my banking. It's embarrassing for me to have Mom doing banking. But I guess responsibility isn't my strong point at the present time.

Love, Mark

On December 28th, Mark transferred to North Iowa Transition Center (NITC) in Mason City, Iowa. There, he acquired a new doctor and psychiatrist.

At times Mark seemed cheerful when I spoke to him on the telephone but was depressed much of the time. He and his grandparents

---

1   "The Waltons" was a television series from 1971-1981

visited each other often. He was able to take his guitar to The Center and began renewing his interest in music. He got a job interviewing people over the telephone but was unhappy and quit. His doctor, not concerned about the job termination, said to me, "It was not Mark's type of employment." Mark continued to do well at The Center, so was fully discharged from MHI in Independence.

CHAPTER 4

Losing Hope, More Hospitalizations, Grandpa Died

1990-1991

AT THE END of January 1990, I received this letter from Mark:

Dear Mom,

I'm sinking fast. I don't have any purpose in my life anymore. At least, before, I always wanted to be something. Now I lay in bed and hate my life.

I don't have any energy or motivation. My guitar instruction books got too hard for me, and I don't have the will to try any harder.

My phone calls to Mark were extremely challenging as I attempted to lift his spirits and motivate him. I would remind him of his past accomplishments, his talents, and his skills. After our conversations, I felt drained.

On February 5th, Mark's cousin Joel from Minneapolis, Minnesota, visited Mark. Mark called and told me, "Joel was unhappy that he could not cheer me up. I feel like sleeping all the time, and my weight is out of control. I have a job interview in the morning, but it only pays $4.00 an hour, so I will probably sleep past the interview, which is at 9:00 a.m."

I encouraged Mark to look forward to the interview because he would be around people with whom he could converse–that it would improve his outlook on life, but he did not attend it.

On April 3rd, Mark was admitted to Mercy Hospital, Mason City, Iowa. He learned about this time that his Grandpa Brown was seriously ill. When Mark was dismissed from the hospital on April 9th, he went to his grandparents' home in Floyd. NITC did not appear to have any special procedures to observe clients upon return from a hospital stay.

On April 16th, Mark returned to NITC, but he was unable to get his Lithium. Two days after I contacted his case manager in Charles City, he finally got it.

On April 20th, 1990, Grandpa Brown died. How traumatic this must have been for Mark.

My Grandpa was a great man who could fix anything. My grandpa was the smartest and toughest guy in the world–and my cousin Joe was with him when he died. Thank you, Joe. The more I learn about my deceased Grandpa, the more I like him. He helped me get my 1954 Chevy Pickup running. He was a trapper. That is when you put something your prey really craves next to your trap. Then you make a map of where you put your traps. Then you go home and eat up all your buttered popcorn while you are kicked back in your easy chair, watching your boob tube. I really miss my Grandpa. I am such a fortunate dog for knowing my Grandpa before he went to heaven. I really don't want to be alive. All I can think of is being at my Grandfather's grave and crying like a baby.

Grandpa's funeral was on April 24th. Mark wrote this poem for his grandfather, which his brother, Kevin, read at the service:

GRANDPA BROWN…
My mind really had to roam
   To write this little poem.
This will do for the time it took
   But to describe Ralph Brown I'd need
To write a book.

He's never been known to do anything wrong
   He likes to work hard all day long.
He doesn't believe in fussin'
   And you rarely catch him cussin'.
He has the ability to think things through
   And you know that his stories are always true.

He's always willing to give you a ride in his boat
   Regardless of all the things he has to tote.
There's not an animal that he can't tame
   And he has never turned one away that was sick or lame.
He raised beautiful animals when I was a boy,
   He did it for everyone to enjoy.
More modest a man you will never meet
   And to spend a day with him is really a treat.
He's been many a place, both near and far,
   But the last place you'll find him is inside a bar.
Beans and corn were his main kind of crop
   And he loves to create things out in his shop.
His wife, Doris, cooks him wonderful meals.
   She has a shiny Cadillac for her set of wheels.

He's never satisfied 'til he gets the job done
   Or when he hears on the news that the Twins have won.
Just a little popcorn at night
   Is all it takes to make him feel just right.
Between him and Ernie there's nothing they can't do.
   They have probably even done something for you.
He built his kids' houses on his own land
   For to do something for them makes him feel most grand.

You'll never catch his nose where it shouldn't belong.
   His ethics and morals are like a well-written song.
Church to him is no big deal.
   Living right to him is real.
In my life he's one of the few
   Who has always been true.

This man that I admire so much
   All of our lives his goodness has touched.
At times this world gets cold and hard
   It's dog-eat-dog out there for sure.
But it's not that way in Grandpa's yard.
   Life here seems good and pure.

I hope the Great Grandkids will find
   The magic of Grandpa's farm
In the years to come
   As well as the years behind.

In May, Mark was returning to his former self. He attended the Iowa AMI (Alliance for the Mentally Ill) State Convention, received a new medication (Prozac), and moved from NITC into an apartment. By June, he had begun working part-time at Sears in Mason City.

In August, I visited Mark at his apartment and at his work. He seemed much improved, though somewhat depressed and pessimistic. He complained of drowsiness and needed to sleep often.

The following month was Grandma Brown's auction. Mark was tremendously helpful in preparing for the sale. He renewed his interest in the restoration of his truck and regularly worked on it at his grandmother's in Floyd.

Mark gave his girlfriend a ring for Christmas and asked her to marry him. She accepted his proposal, and they seemed very happy. They made plans to attend college in Waterloo, Iowa, in August. Mark planned to quit his job at Sears so he could work on his pickup in order to have reliable transportation while attending school. Both were excited about their upcoming plans.

In January 1991, Mark was becoming easily provoked and upset by minor incidents again. He had a disagreement with his grandmother, removed his tools from her garage, and discontinued working on his truck there. He told me that he was having trouble with his fiancée, that he didn't trust her anymore, and that the relationship was off. As a result of his growing aggressiveness, he had pushed her so forcefully her kidney was bruised.

Our telephone conversations were becoming shorter and shorter—to the point that Mark would hang up when he heard my voice.

Due to his erratic behavior, on February 3rd, I called NITC to try and get help for Mark. The staff was unable to locate him. He hadn't shown up for work on February 4th, and his supervisor didn't know where he was. It was evident that Mark was in a downward spiral.

In the early morning of February 5th, Mark kicked in the door to a Charles City bank because he "needed to use the telephone." Because of his behavior, he was taken to MHI by police. The next day he called me and informed me that he had donated his belongings to a charity store in Charles City. Upon my request, the store returned most items; however, his tools and many other items had already been sold.

After a court hearing on February 8, 1991, the decision was made to have Mark committed.

Once again, Kevin went through the familiar motions of dealing with the interruptions in his brother's life: contacting Mark's landlord and releasing his apartment; having his phone disconnected; retrieving and storing his vehicles, computer, and microwave; forwarding his mail to me; and cleaning his apartment.

As part of Mark's treatment, on March 6th, he was transferred from MHI to the University of Iowa Hospital in Iowa City, Iowa, until he returned to MHI on March 20, 1991.

Near the end of his stay, Mark visited his fiancée from March 22nd until March 26th. They resolved their differences, and when Mark was dismissed from MHI on March 28th, they moved back in together. By May, though, the relationship was over; they broke up, and Mark moved into his own apartment.

By June, Mark was slipping fast. Upset over his breakup with his fiancée, his great uncle recognized that Mark was headed for trouble. In Mark's time of crisis, the family networking that took place was absolutely amazing. Relatives, friends, and law enforcement personnel were in minute-by-minute contact with each other. It all began with a telephone call from Great Uncle Elden Pyle and escalated to a stand-off with the state tactical team. After a dramatic confrontation, with Mark fending off law officers from a porch roof in front of a large crowd of spectators, and after being sprayed with Mace, he fell 12 feet to the ground.

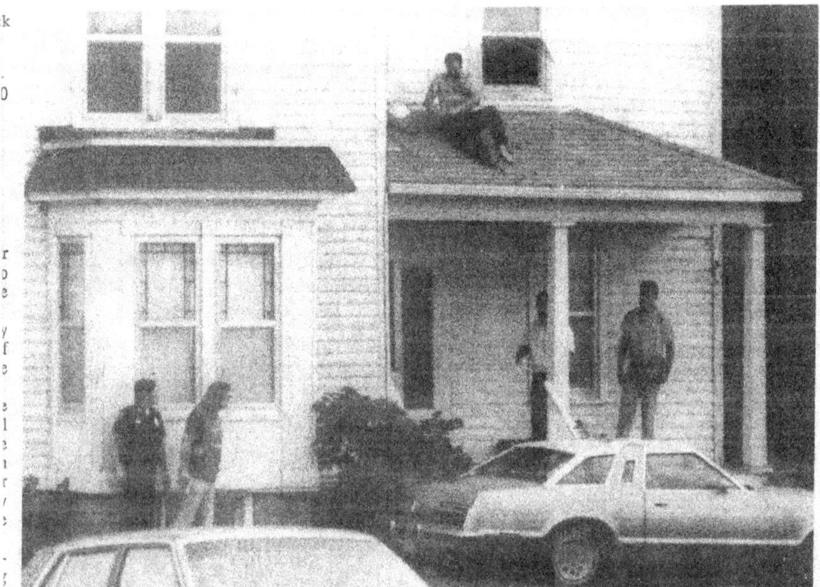

Stand-off

Law enforcement officers try to coax Mark Ostrander down from the roof of a house at 1100 Kelly St. Thursday night. Throwing objects down stairs and out the window, Ostrander held officers at bay for about 90 minutes before falling from the roof and being subdued.

Confrontation with officers

Stand-off ends after 90 minutes

By Mark Wicks

Law enforcement officers from Charles City, Floyd County and the state were held at bay for nearly 90 minutes Thursday evening with threats and acts of violence by a man who was finally subdued after falling from a second-story roof.

Charles City chief of police Paul Scranton reported that officers were called to 1100 Kelly St. at 7:46 p.m. in regard to a disturbance call. When they arrived, they discovered 31-year-old Mark Ostrander rampaging through his upstairs apartment of the two-story house, violently throwing things around the apartment, down the stairs and out the windows.

"He didn't have a weapon that we could see, but he was extremely violent," explained Scranton. "He came downstairs once and had a couple of clubs in hand, threatened the officers and chemical agents were used on him."

At that point, according to Scranton, Ostrander ran back upstairs and held officers at bay by flinging objects down the narrow stairwell.

"There was no way to get up there, so the decision was made to call in the state tactical team," Scranton said.

The Mason City-based district tactical team consists of specially-trained state law officers and is led by Lt. Richard Fellin. The team is trained in dealing with violent standoff and hostage situations.

In this case, Scranton said, local officers were fairly confident from the beginning that Ostrander was the only person in the apartment. He said one occupant was removed from the downstairs right away for safety reasons.

"We determined fairly quickly that he was the only one in the house," the chief reported.

Also while waiting for the tactical team to arrive, police were having a difficult time trying to keep an ever-growing number of bystanders at a safe distance. Brantingham was closed off from Clark St. to North Grand Ave., and the large crowd of spectators pushed back into the NIACC and Pamida parking lots.

Ostrander, meanwhile, continued to throw objects out of the upstairs windows and down the stairs, before finally climbing out of a window and out onto the roof in the front of the house wearing only a pair of pants. He appeared at first to possibly be carrying a rifle, and officers immediately pushed the crowd back even further.

"We thought it might have been a weapon at first, but then determined it appeared to be two table legs or clubs," Scranton explained. "He also had a set of jumper cables."

Ostrander moved about the roof randomly, often tossing more items off the roof, including the jumper cables.

By that time, 10 Charles City police officers were on the scene, as well as four city reserve officers, several

Held at bay

Continued on page 2

Confrontation ends after 90-minute stand-off

Continued from page 1

Floyd County sheriff's deputies and reserves, and the five-man tactical team. A fire engine and ambulance were also called in and asked to stand by.

"He was throwing lit cigarettes about and we were concerned that he might try to burn it down," Scranton said.

"Our biggest concern was to not get any of our officers hurt, and to try and not hurt him. Property can be replaced, but we didn't want anyone hurt if it could be helped."

Tactical team members made an interior assault while officers kept Ostrander talking from inside. During this time, Ostrander appeared to be reacting to the large crowd, especially when he removed his trousers.

"I was very disappointed in the crowd reaction," said Scranton. "They were yelling and egging him on. I was embarassed for the community. This was not a circus. It was not a joke."

A ladder was placed against the roof to try and force Ostrander back in through the window and into the hands of waiting tact team officers, but Ostrander would not bite. He did attack the ladder, however, hitting it with a club and trying to push it away.

Soon afterwards, an officer went up the ladder and threatened Ostrander with more chemical agents. Ostrander at first ran to the corner and covered himself with his arms over his head, then got up and pleaded not to do it, that he was coming down.

A big, reportedly very strong man, Ostrander almost appeared to rush at the ladder and, according to Scranton, was sprayed with the agent. He took one step on the ladder and then fell to the ground.

"He didn't hurt himself in the fall, other than a couple of minor scrapes," Scranton said. "Several officers broke his fall."

Ostrander continued to struggle violently, though, and had to be subdued by a number of officers.

He was then taken to Floyd County Memorial Hospital to be examined, and then was transferred and held on a court order for evaluation.

"We understand he takes medication and it appears he was off of it," Scranton said.

Charges are pending at this time, according to the chief. Several officers, meanwhile, received minor injuries from the falling and thrown debris, much of which was glass which shattered and went flying.

"We were happy to resolve the situation without any serious injury," Scranton said.

CHARLES CITY PRESS

TUESDAY, JUNE 18, 1991

To the editor

Upset over story

I cannot express how disappointed and outraged I was after reading the front page article about Mr. Mark Ostrander in today's issue of your paper. Slow news day?

Don't you think there is a time and place for everything? Obviously not! How humiliating for Mr. Ostrander, his family, and his friends. Isn't it obvious this poor man needed help -- not to have his picture plastered all over the front page of his hometown "newspaper." This was in very poor taste -- how about being a little more sensitive in the future?!

Traci Childers

CHARLES CITY PRESS
TUESDAY, JUNE 25, 1991

To the editor

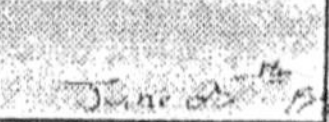

There is help for those who are suffering in silence

I'd like to thank all of the law enforcement personnel who helped save my son's life on Thursday, June 13, during the unfortunate incident when he was on the roof. My son has been battling bi-polar illness for nearly 10 years. He was first stricken in his third year of college at the University of Iowa.

Mental illness is a biological disorder that strikes one out of every four families. It can be devastating and many times tears families apart. Research of diseases of the brain has been far behind that of other biological illnesses, and only recently has help begun to surface for mental illnesses such as bi-polar illness (manic depression), clinical depression, and Haslam-Pinnell Syndrom (schizophrenia).

I am a member of the Dallas Alliance for the Mentally Ill (AMI) which is an affiliate of the National Alliance for the Mentally Ill (NAMI) and the Texas Alliance for the Mentally Ill (TEXAMI). NAMI is a grassroots, self-help support and advocacy organization of families and friends of people with serious mental illnesses. NAMI's mission is to eradicate mental illness and to improve the quality of life for those who suffer from no-fault brain diseases. NAMI is a non-profit, 501(c)(3) corporation, and funds raised are used to benefit seriously mentally ill people and their families. Although I live in Dallas, Texas, June Judge, the past president of Iowa AMI, telephoned me as soon as she learned of Mark's circumstances.

Some Floyd County residents may remember that in 1954 I had the honor of representing Floyd County as their Centennial Queen. Now I feel privileged to be able to inform the citizens who may be suffering in silence that there is help and support for them and their loved ones who have mental illness. Thanks to current research and education of the public, the stigma that has been associated with mental illness is being removed.

Of all 50 states, Iowa is the only state that has a county based funding system for mental illness. Other states that receive federal tax dollars receive matching funds from the federal government, therefore making possible crisis intervention, vocational rehabilitation and social programs. These programs are desperately needed in Iowa.

The Floyd County chairperson for AMI is Neoma Thompson. Please call her at (515) 228-2586. She will be happy to answer your questions and will inform you of AMI activity in your area. Also eager to help are June Judge at (515) 456-2935 and current Iowa AMI President Warren Adams at (515)254-0417.

Colleen Nuncio
Dallas, Texas
(Mother of Mark Ostrander)

Recognizing the need for community-wide awareness

The Alliance for the Mentally Ill (AMI) membership is composed of persons with mental illness, their families, and friends. AMI's obligation is to mentally ill persons and families. AMI actively and constantly works to assure the best possible treatment for mentally ill citizens.

Inaccurate reporting can be very detrimental to those who are mentally ill, as well as to the general mental health of the whole community. Last Thursday KIMT's 10:00 p.m. report left a number of unanswered questions regarding the stand off of the police in Charles City. One of the questions it left was about the manner in which the man who was standing off the police was subdued. Friday's Charles City Press report [Stand-off ends after 90 minutes] almost made one wonder if it were the same event. After talking with several persons I came to the conclusion that the Charles City Press report was fairly accurate.

We are happy that the police officers managed, in a very difficult situation, to keep anyone from getting hurt. We sincerely hope that will continue to be the case in similar circumstances. Chief of Police Scranton said he "was embarrassed for the community" because of the crowd's reaction. From its beginning, the AMI of Floyd County support group has recognized the need for community-wide education regarding mental illness. AMI of Iowa presents programs which could benefit all our citizens. I would like to ask our Chief of Police (and others in our community) to assist in bringing some of these programs to Charles City for our community as a whole. Perhaps then, should there be a similar occurrence, Chief Scranton would not have to be embarrassed.

Concluding, mental illness is a biological illness. We send "Get Well" wishes to our friends who are ill. Our wishes for Mark are that he receive the best of care while hospitalized, that his time in the hospital will pass speedily, and that he will soon be back with his family and friends.

Neoma J. Thompson
For AMI of Floyd County

◼ Editor's Mailbag

Many contributed to Festival success

TO THE EDITOR:

The 53rd Band Festival Committee extends a sincere thank you to the volunteers, participants and spectators for a successful weekend fitting to the tradition of Mason City and Band Festival. The committee owes a large thanks also to the following corporate sponsors that are a major force in a successful Festival:

St. Joseph Mercy Hospital, Bertha Stebens Foundation, Lehigh Portland Cement, Norwest Bank, First Interstate Bank, Globe-Gazette, Park Inn International, Interstate Power Company, Hardee's Restaurants, McDonald's, North Iowa Medical Center, Park Clinic, Liberty Bank, Clear Lake Bank and Trust, The Laird Law Firm, KLSS/KRIB, Optimist Club, Metropolitan Federal Savings, Independent Insurance Agents and Henkel Construction.

Thanks to all of you for making this a weekend of great entertainment and activity.

Mary Hjalmervik
Band Festival Coordinator

Help is available for mentally ill

TO THE EDITOR:

I'd like to thank all of the law enforcement personnel who helped save my son's life on Thursday, June 16, during the unfortunate incident when he was on the roof. My son has been battling bi-polar illness for nearly 10 years. He was first stricken in his third year of college at the University of Iowa.

Mental illness is a biological disorder that strikes one out of every four families. It can be devastating and many times tears families apart. Research of diseases of the brain has been far behind that of other biological illnesses, and only recently has help begun to surface for mental illnesses such as bipolar illness (manic depression), clinical depression, and Haslam-Pinnell Syndrome (schizophrenia).

I am a member of the Dallas Alliance for the Mentally ill which is an affiliate of the National Alliance for the Mentally Ill and the Texas Alliance for the Mentally Ill. NAMI is a grassroots, self-help support and advocacy organization of families and friends of people with serious metnal illnesses. NAMI's mission is to eradicate mental illness and to improve the quality of life for those who suffer from no-fault brain diseases. NAMI is a non-profit corporation, and funds raised are used to benefit seriously mentally ill people and their families. Although I live in Dallas, Texas, June Judge, the past president of Iowa AMI, telephoned me as soon as she learned of Mark's circumstances.

Some Floyd County residents may remember that in 1954 I had the honor of representing Floyd County as their Centennial Queen. Now I feel privileged to be able to inform the citizens who may be suffering in silence that there is help and support for them and their loved ones who have mental illness. Thanks to current research and education of the public the stigma that has been associated with mental illness is being removed.

Of all 50 states, Iowa is the only state that has a county based funding system for mental illness. Other states that receive federal tax dollars receive matching funds from the federal government, therefore making possible crisis intervention, vocational rehabilitation, and social programs. These programs are desperately needed in Iowa.

Eager to answer your questions and inform you of AMI activity in your area are Cerro Gordo Chairperson Terri Kuntz, at 515-424-9648; June Judge at 515-456-2935; and current Iowa AMI President Warren Adams at 515-254-0417.

Colleen Nuncio
Dallas, Texas

An accomplice to genocide

TO THE EDITOR:

I'm sorry, fellow North Iowans, but I beg to differ. Our local National Guard unit was accomplice to an inhumane and unnecessary genocide. Again, the U.S. had to destroy a country in order to save it. In order to "defend" Kuwait, an old-world kingdom of royal families, we fire-bombed 135,000 Iraqi conscripts (forced draftees), their women and children. We also murdered several thousand other civilians in the region to fulfill the Pentagon's 1989 mandate — testing their latest weaponry in combat.

Now, an entire section of the Pentagon has been set up to orchestrate the fanfare of patriotism, yellow-ribboning, TV shows and positive propaganda. Almost as much money is being spent to make our mistake in that distant land look "American" that an equal amount could solve the Kurdish refugee crisis.

Finally, doesn't it occur to anyone that President Bush is allowing those devastating Kuwaiti oil fires to persist, in fact, because it continues to make Hussein look bad and CIA George look good. Bravo to Sen. (Charles) Grassley for not being a party-line fool and for voting against that warfare, which is now proving to taint the image of even Mason City's 1133rd unit.

Billy Rogers
Clear Lake

Opinion Page Policy

Letter of apology

I would like to apologize to Bill Harrold for the way I treated his property.

I would like to apologize to the Charles City Police Dept. and any citizens I may have put in danger.

Thank you.

Mark Ostrander

CHARLES CITY PRESS
TUESDAY, JUNE 25, 1991

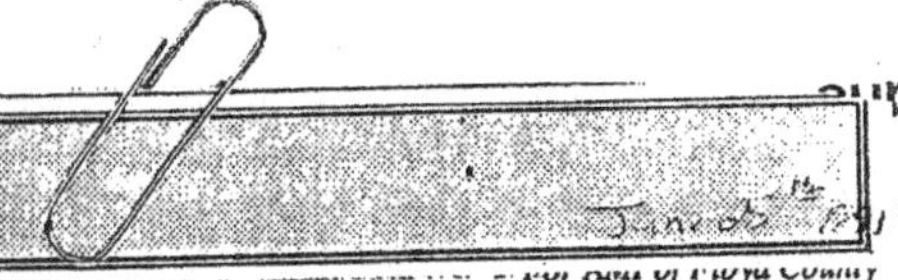

Best wishes for the mental and physical care system

A letter to the Charles City community:.

I wish I could have arrived 90 minutes earlier. I was traveling from Minneapolis and all of the way I knew that this was to be an intense weekend. Our family has been through these "episodes" with Mark many times over the last 10 years. It is difficult to imagine it being like some sort of cage surrounding his thoughts. Kind of like an animal that has been trapped and is willing to chew off its leg rather than remain captured.

I wish there was a place designed for people in these manic stages of their lives -- one would think that there was such a place -- but there isn't any such sanctuary. You see, people like Mark need some place to get help that is in between a state hospital and a half-way house. There is no such place. I know that, you may or may not know that, but most importantly Mark knows that. So when he starts to loose control there really isn't any place to help him through such a crisis. He is justifiably frightened about being institutionalized. I know that when I have visited him in state hospitals I always hated the atmosphere which is negated by the white walls and security doors with the little windows.

I wish that the quality and consistency of care given at these state institutions would be enough to help Mark get better. At least so he could function within a society. I am afraid that this time won't be much different than the past experiences. He will be in there for a few months. They will try to stabilize him with drugs and then he will get out again to fend for himself. The problem is that there is a lot of anger, resentment and stubbornness brewing in Mark. I think that most of us would have anger if we were continually subjected to a system that is basically not effective. Especially if we were literally forced to go.

I wish that Mark didn't have to be taken away again this time the same way as before. I remember being in the police car and hearing over the radio that they had to go and get the leather straps to secure him. When I saw him in the Charles City hospital that night he was handcuffed face down on the cart. He realized he had screwed up and now he was going to be confined once again and drugged to the point of submission.

I wish that where I live wasn't so scary. The night before Mark had drive up to Minneapolis to visit me. I think now that he was reaching out for some sort of help. I gave him what help I could, yet it was not enough. Mark eventually started to get paranoid about the violence that surrounds my neighborhood. It is easy to feel frightened when one comes from a small town in Iowa and all of a sudden you end up in a "crack" neighborhood. I helped Mark get back on the road to Iowa that night, as it was the only place he felt he could be safe. His driving was erratic and I was frightened for his and others' safety. As he drove away I knew that he desperately needed help and it was time that we as a family stood behind him in order to help. That night I called the "crisis hotline" and several other places to no avail. The story for the mentally ill seems to be the same all over (even though Minneapolis prides itself on better health care, that is of course, if you have money). There was nothing else I could do but drive down to Iowa and try to prevent anything from happening.

I wish things were different that night. As soon as I got to Floyd I heard that the police had Mark surrounded and they were trying to get dogs. Dogs! I raced to Charles City going faster than the speedometer could keep up with. When I got there I saw all of these people standing around and making some of the most asinine comments I had ever heard. The police would not let me go near. They were sure that what they were doing was the right thing. I was sure that the least I could do was to talk him back inside out of site of the audience. Mark and I have been able to talk a lot throughout the years and I probably know him better than anybody, yet the police would not take this into any kind of consideration and practically forced me to go stand with the rest of the people. Do you know how terrible it was to see him being "egged" on by some of the people in the crowd -- the amount of immaturity of those people was incredible. And when everybody cheered when Mark fell of the roof and was held down by all of those officers. However, the worst for me was when I saw him strapped down and taken away in the ambulance as I knew what his next few days were going to be like -- white rooms, heavy doors locked, two way mirrors, and drugs that would put down a grizzly.

I wish things could have been different but they aren't. The police did the best job they could. The crowd reactions were natural. Mark acted out the agony over his life the only way he could think of. Our family was as supportive as possible. And the hospital will do what they can for Mark. My only real wish for Mark, for your community, and for our nation as a whole is that we as people become more compassionate towards the strife of mentally ill individuals, by becoming more educated and less judgemental of the actions of others. This will be the only way we can start to dispel some of the myths that surround mental illness. Depression and anxiety is a major part of our American culture and it is time that we as citizens start to recognize instead of deny the emotional traits which are within us all.

Best wishes for your community. Best wishes for Mark. And most of all best wishes to the mental and physical health care system of our country.

Joel Sisson
Minneapolis, Minn.

31

Colleen Nuncio
15151 Berry Trail, #205
Dallas, Texas 75248
214-239-6852

Sunday, July 28, 1991

Hello, Everyone.

It has taken me longer to type this follow-up letter than I anticipated. Busy has been the atmosphere here. As most of you know, Mark is still in the hospital. Grandma and Tina drove Mark to Charles City last week and he spent several days with Tina during a pass from the hospital. I intend to speak with his social worker tomorrow to see what the future holds in store.

Enclosed are a few of the articles that appeared in several newspapers throughout Iowa. Also enclosed are letters to the editors expressing thoughts and opinions of the incident. Joel's letter, especially, brought tears to my eyes. I knew you were an excellent artist, Joel, but I didn't know you were a writer, too!

Everyone has been so supportive and interested in Mark's welfare. Please know that you are appreciated. Mark commented to me during a phone conversation yesterday, that he was watching a television program where the mentally ill were being ridiculed, and he said, "And I'm one of them!" I told him that people do not make fun of someone who has cancer or diabetes, and that is why AMI is working so hard to eliminate the stigma that has been associated with mental illness. I also asked him to please write down the name and time of the program, the television network, and all pertinent information surrounding the statement, because AMI is very effective in positively influencing key people who have the power to promote change.

Love to you all.

Colleen

Sunday, June 16, 1991

Using his powers of observation as well as a great deal of insight, Joel said, "The family networking that took place in Mark's time of crisis is absolutely amazing!"

It all began with a telephone call from Great Uncle Elden Pyle on Saturday, June 8th. Mark had visited Uncle Elden and was obviously upset over his recent break up with Tina. Uncle Elden recognized that Mark was headed for trouble and immediately telephoned

Great Aunt Marie Pyle. Aunt Marie picked up the phone and dialed Mom Colleen in Dallas. Aunt Marie also was concerned about Mark. After passing along the information that Mark may need help, she expressed concern also for Mark's

Grandma Doris Brown who called Dallas to chat. Soon Grandma was aware of the circumstances and her home became the hub of "Operation Mark".

On Tuesday night, June 11th, Friend   , an old schoolmate of Mark's, called to tell

Brother Kevin Ostrander that he was concerned about Mark. Deputy Sheriff Kevin began his own networking with law enforcement personnel.

Wednesday, June 12th,   called Dallas to inform us that Mark was in Minneapolis.

When I arrived home from work, there were messages on my telephone message recorder from Grandma Doris, Aunt Marjorie Sisson, and Cousin Laurie Sisson.

Aunt Marjorie Sisson called to say that Mark had arrived in Minneapolis early that morning. Mark had called Marge at 7:30 a.m. After visiting with Marge, he showered while she pressed his clothes. Then Mark left. Marge hoped Mark would seek out

Cousin Joel Sisson. Joel and Mark did get together, and Joel saw that Mark wasn't thinking clearly. When I called Joel, he informed me that Mark began his way back to Iowa at about 9:15 p.m. Tuesday evening.

Brother Kevin and Friend/Police Officer Mike Niemeyer were in contact with law enforcement agencies along Mark's I-35 route from Minneapolis, Minnesota to Charles City, Iowa.

On Thursday, June 13th, Fiancée   was in touch with Kevin and All were worried about Mark's well-being as they speculated as to his whereabouts.

Sunday, June 16, 1991   Page Two

Thursday evening, June 13th, at 7:46 p.m., Mark's downstairs neighbor called police and reported a terrible commotion coming from Mark's apartment. Mark was tossing items from his second story apartment window. After police arrived, Mark crawled onto the roof, and was uncooperative with the police. Joel drove to Charles City from Minneapolis to see if he could help in any way. Kevin and Friend/Reserve Deputy   kept a vigil from the police station while all others kept in touch by telephone to stay aware of Mark's circumstances. After 90 minutes of encounter, Mark was safely in the ambulance on his way to the hospital.

Kevin is literally his brother's keeper. With the help of Joel, they retrieved what items they could find in the dark, put them into Mark's car and moved them to a safe place.

The next day, Grandma and Joel made a trip to Mark's apartment and Joel cleaned the yard of broken glass while he picked up items remaining from the night before.

The networking continued on to include our extended family of AMI (Alliance for the Mentally Ill) members. As soon as past Iowa AMI President June Judge read of Mark's episode in the Mason City Globe Gazette, she called me to offer her support. As well as making the front page of the Charles City Press and the Mason City Globe Gazette, June informed me that there was an article on the second page of the Des Moines Register. With June's help, I composed letters to the editors of the three newspapers. (Copies enclosed) Chairperson of Floyd County AMI, Neoma Thompson, plans to follow up with letters of her own, and June had already made copies of the Mason City article to mail with a letter to her legislative chairperson.

"THANK YOU" seems hardly enough for the way each and everyone of you played an important part and showed such compassion in Mark's time of need. Please know that you are appreciated.

Love to all of you.

Mom Colleen

MARK'S ADDRESS & TELEPHONE NUMBER:

MARK OSTRANDER
PO BOX 111
INDEPENDENCE IA 50644

(319) 334-2583

RR 2, Box 110
Hampton, Iowa   50441
June 29, 1991

Dear Colleen,

Bless your heart! You are doing so much for the cause
of all people who are coping with a major mental illness.

Neoma has been in touch with you, I know. I haven't seen
the Charles City paper, but she told me the write-up was excellent.
She has two meetings scheduled in addition to meeting with
the cross-agencies. I PRAY, that these leading citizens will
stand firm in a common commitment to more appropriate
services for "our people".

Your letter couldn't have been better!
                she is all you said..and WORSE! She thinks the
label of criminal is preferable to the explanation of the medical
reasons for actions that appear to be without reason.)

accused me of "harassing" her.

Your time-line of family support is a true gem.

Would you mind if I shared that with my daughter, Kate, who is
in the Phd. program at U. of Wisconsin, Madison? She is doing her
thesis on family reaction to their person with mental illness.

"Out of anguish, rises HOPE!"   .

We are now concerned with Mark's ability to find the HOPE in
his so very personal anguish.

Sincerely,

June

Colleen Nuncio
15151 Berry Trail, #205
Dallas, Texas 75248
214-239-6852

Editor
The Des Moines Register
P.O. Box 957
Des Moines, Iowa 50304

Dear Sir:

I'd like to thank all of the law enforcement personnel who helped save my son's life on Thursday, June 16th, during the unfortunate incident when he was on the roof. My son has been battling bi-polar illness for nearly ten years. He was first stricken in his third year of college at the University of Iowa.

Mental illness is a biological disorder that strikes one out of every four families. It can be devastating and many times tears families apart. Research of diseases of the brain has been far behind that of other biological illnesses, and only recently has help begun to surface for mental illnesses such as bi-polar illness (manic depression), clinical depression, and Haslam-Pinnell Syndrome (schizophrenia).

I am a member of the Dallas Alliance for the Mentally Ill (AMI) which is an affiliate of the National Alliance for the Mentally Ill (NAMI) and the Texas Alliance for the Mentally Ill (TEXAMI). NAMI is a grassroots, self-help support and advocacy organization of families and friends of people with serious mental illnesses. NAMI's mission is to eradicate mental illness and to improve the quality of life for those who suffer from no-fault brain diseases. NAMI is a non-profit, 501(c)(3) corporation, and funds raised are used to benefit seriously mentally ill people and their families. Although I live in Dallas, Texas, June Judge, the past president of Iowa AMI, telephoned me as soon as she learned of Mark's circumstances.

Some Floyd County residents may remember that in 1954 I had the honor of representing Floyd County as their Centennial Queen. Now I feel privileged to be able to inform the citizens who may be suffering in silence that there is help and support for them and their loved ones who have mental illness. Thanks to current research and education of the public the stigma that has been associated with mental illness is being removed.

Of all 50 states, Iowa is the only state that has a <u>county</u> based funding system for mental illness. Other States that receive <u>federal</u> tax dollars receive matching funds from the federal government, therefore making possible crisis intervention, vocational rehabilitation, and social programs. These programs are desperately needed in Iowa.

Eager to answer your questions and inform you of AMI activity in your area are Iowa AMI Executive Director Margaret Stout at (515) 254-0417, current Iowa AMI President Warren Adams at (515) 254-0417 and June Judge at (515) 456-2935.

Sincerely,

Colleen Nuncio

Colleen Nuncio
15151 Berry Trail, #205
Dallas, Texas 75248
214-239-6852

August 5, 1991

Dear Tina,

Mark asked me if I would mail this letter to you. He was afraid that you would return his letter unopened if he mailed it directly to you.

I am so sorry that you and Mark have had such misfortune. I know how difficult it is to try to cope with Mark's illness, and I think that you have been tremendous through these bad times. Hopefully, through research, more effective medication and even a cure will soon be forthcoming.

Mark and I have had some in depth conversations recently, and even though he has treated you badly, he thinks the world of you. (We all do, for that matter.)

Will you call me (collect) when you receive this letter and let me know how you are doing? I look forward to hearing from you.

Lots of love,

Colleen

Mark's girlfriend stayed in touch with me throughout Mark's "meltdown." In a letter dated July 10th, she told me that they were getting back together. "Different rules this time. He said he trusts me and that he believes I've been faithful, so I'm hoping that things are going to work out for us."

While he was in the hospital, on August 28th, Mark wrote this letter to her:

In your letter, you said I am full of anger and hate. And right now you couldn't be more right. But this isn't the only Mark you've known. Remember the happy Mark who was living with you and working and fixing things on the truck and the house? That was a happy Mark, a content Mark, a peaceful Mark, a Mark full of hope and dreams. We were shaping a future and shaping it together. Do you remember how important it was for me to get Molly off her chain? When we were young, Grandpa kept all kinds of animals in cages for people to enjoy (squirrels, foxes, raccoons, deer, crows, owls, possums, and others). At first, I thought how great it was to have these animals. Then the more I watched my favorite animals (the raccoons), I noticed that they would chew through a 2 x 4 to get free. They spent their life trying to get free. I used to spend hours in the cage with them, enjoy them, and feeling sorry for them at the same time. Then the first time I was ever locked up, I went berserk, and they had to tie me down. Now, every time I get locked up, I feel like one of those 'coons trying to chew his way out to freedom. At that time, I made a vow to myself that I would never own a dog if I had to keep it on a chain or in a cage.

Isn't it easy to see the difference in Molly when she's on the chain and off? On the chain, she is like a wild, mad dog except to you and me because she knows we'll let her off. When she is off the chain, she is 100% more friendly, a healthier and happier dog.
The hospital is my chain.

There is a big difference between you and me. When you get real mad, you don't say anything—because you know you might regret it later. I don't know where you learned that, but it is a smart thing to know.

Like I said, I'm different when I get mad—I don't take the time to think about what I say. Over and over in my bed, I say to myself, "God, I wish I could take that back, whenever I say something stupid to you. What is so terrible is that I know I can't.

The reason I was so pushy with the wedding was because of how badly I wanted it. I am used to things going to shit in my life, and it was like a race to get it done before anything got fucked up.

Well, __ was a bitch to me, and instead of ignoring her, I thought it was up to me to put her in her place, and it backfired in my face—I didn't get my next pass—that made it impossible to set our date—that put more burden on you and everything got fucked up.

Then you got to see me in my cage, knowing I couldn't get out to spend the weekend planning our wedding and making love to you. All because of some blond that used more hairspray than I use milk.

Remember when we left Molly off at the vet in that little cage? That's what it's like to me when I see you leave me here.

I know that your friends and family are telling you to trash me, but they don't know me like you do.

We've been good to each other and don't stab each other in the back. There aren't too many people around who can understand that kind of a relationship. When I say "stab in the back," I should really use the words "use each other." We've never done that.

I have tried to take the loneliness out of your life and found that you took it out of mine.

We agree on so many things and disagree on so few that we need to focus more on the things we agree on, not the things we don't.

__, my love for you is like a river, and you're asking me to turn it off like a faucet. You make me feel human. You're not only my fantastic lover, but you are my best friend.

You are a ray of light into my life, and without that ray, my life is dark. Please open your heart and let a little bit of that light back into my life, it's so lonely without you.

Love,

Mark

Four months later, on October 9, 1991, Mark was transferred to Country Meadows, Inc., in Webster City, Iowa. Grandma Brown visited Mark there and said it was awful–like an old people's county home–no motivation, no privacy, no anything! Two-thirds of the residents there were mentally ill, and one-third were mentally retarded. Mark's case manager saw that he needed to be in a different atmosphere and tried to get him transferred. Mark was to have his first outpatient therapy with a psychiatrist and counselor three weeks after he arrived.

Mark's court hearing was scheduled for November 12, 1991. When I asked a Country Meadows staff person for a contact in case of emergency, she informed me that no phone numbers could be given out. Mark's case manager was unable to be in court, so they would check on the availability of a Floyd County advocate.

Arraignment was at 9:00 a.m. at the Floyd County Courthouse in Charles City. Mark was taken to the courthouse by Country Meadows staff. June Judge, president of Iowa Alliance for the Mentally Ill (AMI), was in attendance. When I spoke with her, she mentioned how unsavory the staff person's appearance was. "Mark looked better than him." Also attending were AMI member Neoma Thompson, AMI client Paul G, and the public defender. Mark became upset when mental illness was mentioned and was not receptive to any help from AMI.

Because Country Meadows' main contact received the letter regarding Mark's hearing too late, his legal counsel was not there. The arraignment was to be continued on February 4, 1992. The trip to Charles City was for nothing.

On November 17, 1991, I sent this letter to Mark.

Dear Mark,

I know you think about your future: what you will do and where you will go when you leave Webster City.

You mentioned to me that you feel it will be difficult for you to get a job in the cities where you have lived because of stigma and prejudice.

There is a career waiting for a person with precisely your experience in a field where you are desperately needed. And there are no limits to advancement. You can begin at the local level and move to the state and national level if you so desire. With your education, knowledge, background, and experience, I know you are qualified for the position.

You will work with people whose level of thinking rises above the prejudice and stigma about which you have been concerned. Among these people are well-educated, capable individuals in a wide variety of professions and occupations, including medicine, education, law, art, and business.

One of the requirements for this position, in order to achieve the necessary goals, is a great deal of <u>compassion for people and a willingness to represent others</u>. I have observed these qualities in you many times and know you possess these prerequisites.

You will need to be a spokesperson—not unlike the legislators who represent you in government. You will be respected, and people will listen to what you have to say…because you will have first-hand experience of your topic. You have been there. You are an authority on the subject.

I know you are qualified for many lines of work and whatever you pursue is your choice. I believe you will be more deeply satisfied and acquire a greater sense of fulfillment with a position that offers purpose and meaning to your life—one that adds a sense of pride and accomplishment—and one in which you are able to attain the high ideals that are so much a part of you.

You can realize your goals, Mark. The support and cooperation of other people is needed to achieve any worthwhile goal. Please know that you have support from people with a reservoir of knowledge, education, and information for you to draw upon. Please know, too, that these people will be there to share important information with you when you need them.

You have an opportunity to lend credibility to your reactions to a hospital/living situation that was and is inefficient and ineffectual: lack of professional contact, insufficient staff, delay or lack of supportive counseling, and inappropriate environment for individual recovery (living conditions which delay rather than promote recovery). You also have the opportunity to do something to correct a bad situation—yours and thousands of others who have been and are being discriminated against at this very moment.

Love, Mom

CHAPTER 5

One Step Forward, Two Steps Back

January 1992–May 1994

ON JANUARY 13, 1992, Mark was able to transfer to the Center for Personal Development (CPD) in Ames, Iowa. At this transitional housing program, he had the opportunity to transition back into society and lead a normal lifestyle. I was in contact with the staff from the beginning. By March, I was able to speak with Mark. When I called him, he sounded glad to hear from me and asked lots of questions about the family and me. He was not happy after meeting with his doctor for the first time, as the doctor's only suggestion to combat fatigue was to "take naps." Added to his medications Lithium and Tegretol, were Klonopin and Haldol.

Early in April, Mark sent this letter to his family:

Hello,

I'm trying to turn over a new leaf and actually write my relatives. Grandma helped me update my addresses, so now I'm ready to roll. My address is 1008 Burnett, Ames, IA 50010. So many

times thoughts of all of you cross my mind. If you get the chance, jot me down a few lines, and tell me what is going on in your lives.
Catch ya later, Mark

"Catch ya later" was a phrase that Mark used often. When I read that phrase in his letter, it brought back memories of happy times.

Mark shared a special bond with his Aunt Marge. In a letter to her dated June 15, 1992, he wrote of his deepest thoughts and feelings. "I'm trying my best to get a handle on life. Uncertainty is my biggest enemy. Fear of being caught in a ho-hum job is another."

Although Mark worked hard to comply with the requisites of the program at CPD, he became unstable and was admitted to the Iowa Lutheran Hospital from July 24th to August 4th, 1992.

Mark completed the program and graduated from CPD on April 5, 1993. He began employment as a volunteer computer technician for the Ames Public School System. He did well and took pride in his work. He also worked at Arby's fast food restaurant but was working so many hours that he had to pay back his Medicare Insurance at $50.00 per month. In this letter to his brother, Kevin (Oz), it was obvious how fervently Mark was trying to stay on top of his life.

OZ

I am sitting here in my new hangout, the Ames Public Library Media Center. This afternoon I am working on a Macintosh LC II, system 7.0.1, with 4 Megabytes of RAM and a 16 Megabyte Hard drive. I am utilizing an Apple Personal Laserwriter and working with Microsoft Word 4.0.

Thanks for letting me look around at the equipment in the Comm. Center, I thought that was really exciting. Cables, monitors, computers, and radios fascinate me. The other night in the Comm. Center you asked me if I knew about fonts. I thought I would give you a few examples of some of the more common ones. *A font is a style of print, like* **Chicago***, or* `courier`*, or* Geneva*, or* Helvetica*, or* London *or* Monaco*, or* New York*, or times. I have also included the sheet named Test Document. I printed this at Apple headquarters in Dallas while attending Laser Printer training school.*

Oz, an average week, I spend 25 hours at one job, 15 hours of Volunteer work (repaying my debt to the taxpayers), 5-10 hours using the computer at the library, 15 to 20 hours of home study. I rarely watch TV, and I even more rarely go up town. I am 110% committed to my career. I do this with a severely impaired sleep pattern due to taking more than 80 pills a week. If you think l can try harder, please, tell me what I can do, then give me the time and date, and I will try and fit it into my schedule.

Included is the career information I mentioned. The first three pages labeled Contents, is the table of contents for the Dictionary of Occupational Titles, found in most libraries. The book has a small explanation of each occupation. The Career choices at DMACC has some interesting information in it and also a neat little world-of-work map on the back that might help you to narrow your career choices. I also sent you the results of my Strong Vocational Interest Test for a laugh.

This magazine caught my eye, and I just knew it would bring saliva to your mouth. Now don't run out and buy a Ruger Mini-14 5.56mm unless I can target practice with it, too.

Say hello to the BIG 0 and the little bitty o for me.

Mark

Mark was hospitalized twice more in 1993. He became unstable in June and once again in December. On December 30th, law enforcement officers took Mark to Iowa Lutheran Hospital when he was found standing in the median of a busy highway. He was admitted to a secured area of the hospital. Police found Mark's apartment locked and his car there. When I spoke with Mark, he sounded very groggy. His doctor told me that Mark was fatigued. By January 2, 1994, Mark was transferred from the secured area of the hospital to the non-secured area.

After his discharge from Iowa Lutheran Hospital in mid-January, Mark was afraid he would be unable to get any more medication, so he was "conserving" his meds. I spoke with the pharmacy owner about Mark's pharmacy bill. He placed Mark on a pricing program that priced his prescription at near-pharmacy cost.

On January 17, 1994, Mark went to Omaha to see his stepfather. The next day, he drove back to Ames in a snowstorm, even after his dad asked him to stay. On the 19th, a CPD staff member drove Mark to Mary Greely Hospital in Ames because Mark became paranoid. He had open sores on his face. (Could it be frostbite?) Later it was learned that Mark had tried to straighten his teeth with a power grinding tool.

From January 20 through February 15, 1994, Mark remained in Iowa Lutheran Hospital, where he had been transferred from Mary Greely Hospital. In early February, his doctor said that if Mark didn't improve, he might need to transfer him to Cherokee State Hospital. By the 15th, Mark had improved and moved back to CPD. On February 17th, he moved into an apartment in Ames. By March 7th, he moved to yet another apartment because he said his neighbors were continually playing loud music.

After being turned away by several dentists because they would not accept Medicare, he made an April 5th appointment with a dentist to whom he paid $200.00 before any work was done. Mark asked the dentist specifically to repair his top four front teeth that he had attempted to straighten with his power grinder. After the dentist had x-rayed, cleaned, and filled several teeth (none of which included the requested repair), he told Mark he could do nothing more for him. I was outraged, because Mark had told this dentist about his finances and his limited schedule. Rather than honor Mark's request, the office did not offer appointments that would allow him to get his crowns repaired. After speaking with a representative from Iowa Medical Services, I learned that most office employees don't understand their patients' Medicare, Medicaid, or Title IXX funding.

Mark called me on April 4, 1994, lonely and depressed. I called the Director of Ames AMI to see if there was a Compeer Program[2] in effect. I was put in touch with an AMI member, "M," a retired microbiologist, who subsequently visited Mark. He told me that Mark's apartment was clean and that Mark was personable and amiable. They had a good conversation, and M suggested they attend a ballgame sometime.

On April 22nd, Mark came to his grandmother's while I was visiting her. He seemed quite depressed. After returning to Ames, he called me when I was at his brother Kevin's house. He said he "just wanted to talk."

After I returned to Dallas, Mark called me and discussed his dental work. He was discouraged about money and hung up without telling me good-bye. I called Mark's new dentist, who accepted Medicare/Medicaid, and learned patients were allowed two crowns per year. The dentist approved Mark's paying over a period of time; Mom and I agreed to share the cost of additional crowns.

In May, I called M. He said he planned to visit Mark again.

Mark called and updated me on his dental work progress and told me that his doctor prescribed methylphenidate to combat his drowsiness and fatigue.

Mid-May, Mark attended a Manic Depressive support group

---

2   Compeer Program is a program that matches adults in the community who are in recovery from mental illness with a volunteer friend. One-to-one matches spend about 4 hours together per month, engaging in activities such as going for a walk, getting a cup of coffee, or watching a sporting event.

meeting in Des Moines. The next day, he called and said that he was waking up feeling panicky, and it felt like he had pressure on his brain, which strong aspirin sometimes helped relieve. He had also been reading about manic depressive illness and mentioned the high rate of suicide among persons with manic depression.

Mark told me, "I don't want to live anymore. I can only function about four hours a day and am spending most of my time in bed."

I replied, "Mark, why don't you give it one more try? Come to Dallas, and we will see if we can get your meds adjusted, improve your life, and give you a reason to live." He agreed to come and would arrive May 28, 1994.

CHAPTER 6

Return to Dallas, Persistent Efforts, Suicide Attempt

May 26, 1994–December 27, 1994

WHILE WAITING FOR Mark to arrive, I searched for a psychiatrist. I contacted several psychiatrists and learned their fees were much too high, and they did not accept Medicare. I finally was able to make an appointment with Dr. H, who accepted Medicare and agreed to meet with Mark on an outpatient basis.

Mark arrived in Dallas on May 28th. He and I attended a free public forum on medication for mental illness at the University of Texas Southwestern Medical Center. Mark slept through most of the 2-hour meeting.

After meeting with Dr. H on June 1st, Mark consented to go into the hospital. Arrangements were made to admit Mark into Green Oaks Hospital on Monday, June 6, 1994. On the day of his admission, Green Oaks would not accept Mark as a patient, so Dr. H said he would see if he could get him into Presbyterian Hospital's sleep disorder clinic. Another office appointment was set for Wednesday, June 8th.

On the 8th, Dr. H called and canceled Mark's appointment. He indicated that, unless Mark went to the emergency room saying he was suicidal, it would be nearly impossible to refer Mark to someone for immediate hospitalization. If he claimed to be suicidal, he would then be accepted as a patient and could get into the sleep disorder clinic at Presbyterian for consultation. He would also be treated for his depression and his inability to sleep at night. Dr. H also suggested alternative treatments, including different medication – Depakote or Risperidone – and electroconvulsive therapy.

Dr. H said he would look at Presbyterian Hospital's on-call schedule and recommended that Mark go to the ER when his colleague was taking calls. With Medicare, he would be admitted. Dr. H stated that he hated to be manipulative in order to get anything accomplished, and he would rather I did not tell Mark.

Dr. J would be on call Tuesday, June 21, 1994, from 5 p.m. until 7 a.m., and on Sunday, June 26th, all day. He would see Mark in the ER, then make an appointment to see him. But when I discussed the plan with Mark, he disagreed and decided not to follow through.

My last contact with Dr. H was June 16th when I telephoned him; he said he was unable to talk, and he asked to call me back. I never heard from him again.

Four days later, I stopped at Dr. H's office. There would be no hospitalization. His assistant returned my original check, saying there was an overcharge. His office would file for Medicare and reimbursement for Mark's appointments.

Dr. H tried his very best to get treatment for Mark. Due to the lack of health insurance, his hands were tied. I sent him this letter to show my appreciation:

July 13, 1994

Dear Dr. H,

Thank you so much for your many attempts to help my son, Mark Ostrander. Please know that your efforts are appreciated.

It can be very frustrating when you are attempting to admit a patient into a hospital without success. I'm looking forward to that time when we will not encounter so many dead ends.

Last week I attended the NAMI Convention in San Antonio. This annual convention of the National Alliance for the Mentally Ill initiates many changes in our society, and it gave me the inspiration (even more than I have now) to "get something done!"

Enclosed is a copy of one of the letters that I wrote to my congressman after attending the convention. It is one of many written (there were approximately 1,600 registered attendees at the convention) and I hope we can get help in treating your profession equally regarding health insurance.

After much discussion and searching, Mark is getting help from Dr. J. Mark has decided to move to Dallas, and with our support, we are looking forward to a happier and more meaningful life for him.

Thank you again for your understanding. If I can help you in any way, please don't hesitate to call me.

Sincerely,
Colleen Nuncio, Secretary Dallas AMI

Dear Senator:

After attending the annual convention for the National Alliance for the Mentally Ill (NAMI) in San Antonio, Texas, this weekend, I was excited to learn of the new medications that have been developed for persons with mental illness. A high percentage of persons with mental illness have a positive response to the drugs and are able to return to their active roles in society. This will save our government millions of dollars each year and eliminate the "revolving door syndrome" of repeated hospitalizations.

Persons with mental illness must have access to medical care, and these new medications before any benefit can be realized.

Of the approximately 1,600 registered attendees at our convention, we all shared one concern. There is no parity in health insurance for persons with mental illness.

Please help us to create a bill for universal health coverage and support our need for parity in health insurance.

Thank you.

Sincerely,

Colleen Nuncio, Secretary Dallas Alliance for the Mentally Ill

On June 21, 1994, Mark and I found help when Dr. J accepted Mark as a patient. I told Dr. J that he was Mark's last resort. We presented copies of current medications and the following symptoms:

1) Severe daily headaches. "Weird, pressure feeling."
2) Total fatigue. Cannot function over 4 hours without sleep. This may vary from 2 to 6 hours.
3) No motivation.
4) Methylphenidate benefits last for 2 hours maximum, during which time Mark feels energetic and motivated. Does not last. When he takes the medicine, after 2 hours, he is overtaken by drowsiness. If he takes more, no benefits. Needs to sleep.

Dr. J changed Mark's medication from generic methylphenidate to Ritalin because he said it was more potent and effective. Mark seemed to improve with his new medication regimen. His attitude was upbeat, and he rekindled a prior relationship with an old girlfriend with whom he spent a great deal of time. Mark's grandmother purchased a

1984 pickup truck for him, and he became interested in its upkeep. He played tennis, attended family get-togethers, and began to look for a job.

By July, Mark decided to stay in Dallas, at my invitation, so he drove his pickup to Ames, Iowa, to get his belongings from his apartment and store his furniture. Because Mark's medical bills were too high for his social security income, he would need to get into the DCMHMR (Dallas County Mental Health and Mental Retardation) system.

In August Mark got a job with Target Stores. Although happy with his job, the relationship with his girlfriend deteriorated to the point where it was nearly nonexistent, adding to his feelings of low-esteem.

Mark became obsessed with his job, carrying a notebook with him and recording every detail. Each day after work, he drove to a quiet park and reviewed the day's events. He entered job responsibilities and plans in his notebook. He was sleeping less and less and stayed out all night, arriving home early in the morning.

On September 1st, I convinced Mark to go to Dr. J's office, as he was becoming unstable. Dr. J and his assistant drove Mark from his office directly to Baylor Richardson Hospital; he was hospitalized there until Friday morning, September 9th, at 9:40 a.m.

At 7 o'clock that evening, Mark went to work at Target. He arrived home at 6 o'clock the following morning and went directly to bed. He arose at 8 a.m., ran errands, returned home, slept for a half-hour, then went to work at Target at 4 p.m.

On September 11th, Mark told me that he had slept two hours in his truck in Lynn's driveway. Later, Mark's cousin, Denise, called me and stated that Mark had arrived at her house early that morning. She commented to Mark that it was ironic that he could not stay awake before, and now he was unable to sleep. Mark responded, "Isn't that good!" Mark slept at her house from 10 a.m. until 3 p.m. She remarked that it sounded as though Mark was vomiting in the bathroom after he quickly excused himself from the table at lunch. Mark took his meds (except his sleeping pills) and left at 5 p.m.

At 7:45 p.m., Mark called to tell me that he was going to visit Lynn. He arrived at her house at 8:45 p.m. Lynn observed that he was hyperactive and could not concentrate or focus on the conversation. Although Mark wanted to sit in his truck in her driveway to do paperwork, Lynn convinced him to sit on her patio instead. She said he smoked incessantly and laughed inappropriately.

Mark arrived home on September 12th at 7 a.m. He accidentally set off the security alarm, telling me later that it was broken. In fact, he had not been able to remember the code. When he announced he was going to play tennis, I suggested he sleep first, but he wouldn't talk to me. He remembered his doctor's appointment: "Yes, one o'clock," he replied when I asked. When I left for work at 7:30 a.m., he was in the parking lot with his tennis racquet. I called Dr. J and talked to him about Mark's actions. He advised me to get him to the hospital.

I arrived home from work at 8:30 p.m. Mark had slept from 3:40 p.m. until 7:40 p.m. and had piled all of his belongings, including his clothing and books, in the middle of his room. He transferred some items to his truck and put others neatly in his closet and on shelves. When he left at 10 p.m., his face was puffy, and his eyes were bulging. Later, Dr. J's assistant called and asked if Mark could spend the night with Lynn, his sister. I told him that was not an option.

At 7 o'clock the next morning, Lynn's husband, who worked at Huffine's Chevrolet in Lewisville, saw Mark there having the oil changed in his truck. Co-workers said Mark would not respond unless he was touched. To pay for the service, Mark threw money on the counter and said, "Take what you need."

At 11 a.m., I called Dr. J's office and asked if Mark had come in for his appointment. He had not.

Later that evening, around 5 p.m., Mark knocked on our door, unable to get the door unlocked, even though he had a key. Martin could see that Mark had not slept for a long time and tried to convince him to go to the hospital. After a lengthy conversation, Mark agreed to go, but only if Dr. J's assistant would take him. That evening, the Assistant drove Mark to Baylor Richardson Medical Center, where Mark was re-admitted.

During his hospitalization, I tried to find housing for Mark. To qualify for transitional housing, he needed to be in the DCMHMR System and needed a doctor referral. After numerous unsuccessful attempts to contact the Routh Street clinic, I finally received help from the director of DCMHMR. He asked me to document the events prior to my phone call to him. Following is the letter that I sent to the director.

September 16, 1994
Mr. (Director),
Dallas County Mental Health and Mental Retardation
1341 W. Mockingbird, #1000E
Dallas, TX 75247
Dear Mr. (Director):

Thank you for helping me to get a response from the Routh Street Clinic after my many efforts to communicate with that facility failed. Following is a summary of my son's situation and what led to my unsuccessful attempts to communicate with the Routh Street Clinic staff.

When my son, Mark, moved to Dallas May 28, 1994, he was suicidal. He was unemployed and on Social Security and Medicare. During the month of June, I paid over $300 for medication and doctor bills. In July, I set an appointment to get Mark back into the system due to the high cost of his medical bills.

8/3/94: Intake Interview with __. Set appointment for psychiatric evaluation with Dr. ___ for 9/6/94 at 2:00 p.m.

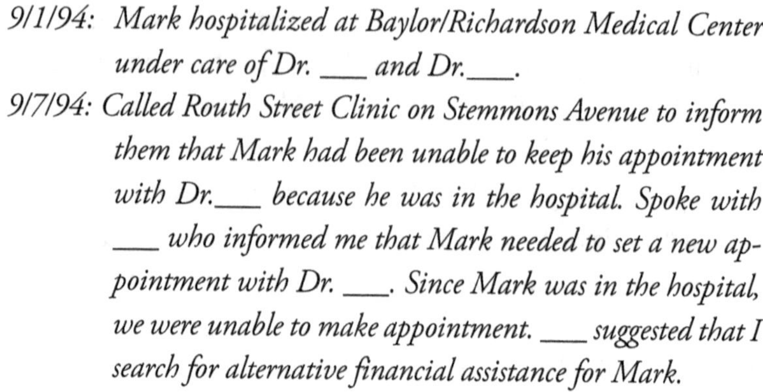

9/1/94: Mark hospitalized at Baylor/Richardson Medical Center under care of Dr. ___ and Dr.___.

9/7/94: Called Routh Street Clinic on Stemmons Avenue to inform them that Mark had been unable to keep his appointment with Dr.___ because he was in the hospital. Spoke with ___ who informed me that Mark needed to set a new appointment with Dr. ___. Since Mark was in the hospital, we were unable to make appointment. ___ suggested that I search for alternative financial assistance for Mark.

I called several agencies seeking financial assistance for Mark including the Community Council of Greater Dallas, the Social Security Administration, Medicare/Medicaid, Information and Referral for Social Services, and United Way. Some of the agencies were able to help if Mark was in the DCMHMR system.

9/8/94: At the suggestion of a member of Dallas AMI, I spoke with Intake Coordinator (IC) of the Phoenix House to seek housing for Mark. I learned that Mark needed to be in the DCMHMR system to qualify for housing at that facility, and IC asked that I have Mark's DCMHMR caseworker call him.

I called Routh Street Clinic and asked for the name of Mark's caseworker, as Mark had lost this information during the turbulence of his hospital admittance. No one seemed able to locate Mark's caseworker, although I thought Mark had written the case worker's name in his appointment book along with his doctor's name. When I asked to speak with the person who held Mark's initial interview, I was told she no longer worked there. I asked that a caseworker or Supervisor please call me.

9/9/94: Mark was dismissed from Baylor/Richardson Medical Center.

9/13/94: Mark was re-hospitalized at Baylor Richardson. I called Routh Street Clinic and told the intake coordinator my dilemma. I asked him to personally ask Miss ___ to call me.

9/14/94: I called Routh Street Clinic and asked to speak with Dr. ___. I learned that he was out of the clinic on Wednesday, so I called his private practice office and left a message for him to call me. He returned my call Wednesday evening at which time I informed him of Mark's situation. Dr. ___ informed me that he knew Dr. ___ and could communicate with him. He suggested that I call ___, but I informed him that she would not return my calls. Dr. ___ then suggested that I ask IC to set Mark's doctor appointment.

9/15/94: I called IC to set an appointment with Mark's doctor. She informed me that Mark would have to have another intake interview since he "left the system." I explained to her that Mark had not left the system, but had been hospitalized before he had a chance to meet with his doctor. At that time, she asked me to hold the line. I held and held. When no one came back on the line, I hung up.

Later, I spoke with the records department to see if Mark's records could be located. After putting me on "hold" for a long time, she asked me for my telephone number, as "someone will have to call you." I said, "No, that's okay. I'll call Director."

That was when I called you and told you about my problem. Shortly after I called you, IC called me. I asked her if she had spoken with you, and she replied she had not. I told her that you would be getting in touch with her.

By late afternoon, I received a second call from IC. She apologized for not getting back with me, and assured me that Mark's needs would be met.

Thanks again for your help. I appreciated your follow up call on Friday morning, September 16, and was happy to be able to report to you that progress had been made. If I can help you in any way, please call me.

Sincerely,

Colleen Nuncio,

Secretary Dallas AMI

On September 20, 1994, Mark was placed on a one- to two-month waiting list for housing at a transitional center for persons with mental illness. An appointment was made to meet with the manager of Phoenix House on Tuesday, September 27th, at 11:00 a.m.

When I visited Mark at Baylor Richardson after work, he asked me to leave. He also told me that he called the Target store where he worked and quit his job–because "I can't get along with my supervisor."

Mark was discharged from the hospital on September 21st at 5 p.m. The doctor told me that Mark was just smoking cigarettes, flirting with the nurses, and was not cooperating in groups. He also said that Mark had a strong, clear plan and was adamant about going home. The next day, the doctor called to tell me that Mark did not have his medication and "will probably deteriorate quickly." Mark didn't have medication at home, as the doctor thought; in fact, he had left it at Dr. J's office when the Assistant took him to the hospital. At 12:30 p.m., Mark was in Dr. J's office and in a daze. The doctor went to get the medication, but when he came back, Mark was gone and did not come back until late that afternoon. He took his meds in the office and told the staff that he would be staying at the Salvation Army that night.

At 6:15 p.m., Mark called his sister from a pool hall, letting her know that he had a doctor's appointment the next day. Ending the conversation with "I love you," Lynn thought that was odd, as they did not usually end their conversations in that manner.

After no contact with Mark for two days, I filed a Missing Person Report. A police officer went to Target and looked through Mark's employee files, then searched for Mark's truck at Alpha and Montfort without success. At 6:00 o'clock Saturday evening, I canceled the Missing Person Report when Mark arrived home.

Monday morning, Dr. J's office called me. Mark was in their office. Dr. J said that Mark was one step away from being eligible for commitment and that I needed to get him to Parkland Emergency.

I left work to pick up Mark from Dr. J's office. By the time I arrived, Mark was gone. I drove from the office toward our home and saw him in his truck, entering the street that I was traveling. When I was able to get his attention, I asked him to come home, but he said, "Let's go have breakfast." We went to Denny's Restaurant in Plano, where his friend was working. We sat at a booth, but Mark became upset when I told him I could not give him any money and got up to leave. He agreed to ride in my car with me, and, as we drove, I told him that Dr. J wanted him to go to Parkland. That upset him, and he demanded, "Stop the car and let me out right now!" He began to open the door, even though we were traveling too fast for him to get out. As soon as I could safely move the car to the side of the street, I stopped the car, and he got out and began walking back to the restaurant where his truck was. I followed slowly in my car, staying out of his sight where he would not see me. After Mark went into the restaurant, I returned to Dr. J's office.

Back in Dr. J's office, his assistant told me that I needed to get an order for protective custody so the police could pick up Mark and take him to Parkland Psychiatric Intensive Care Unit. I completed the application and addendum, which the court needed by 4:00 p.m. However, the judge did not sign it because there was missing information on the doctor's certificate. Later, it was decided that the medical review at Parkland could be bypassed. That evening Mark stayed with his friend and her family. When I called her at work the next day, she told me that Mark was "really out of it." Between 10:00 a.m. and 3:00 p.m., Mark had been at his doctor's office, the Phoenix House and Routh Street Clinic. He had telephoned his grandma in Iowa asking for money; earlier, Dr. J's assistant had given Mark $2.00 for gas.

The next morning Grandma called again. Mark was getting a cab from a Shell Station at Campbell and Central (his truck was parked at Baylor Richardson Medical Center) and was on his way to Huffine's in Lewisville to see Curt, his brother-in-law. He arrived around 9:30 a.m. with no money to pay the $40 cab fare, so Curt paid.

Concerned about Mark's behavior, I called the Lewisville Police to see if they could detain Mark until the OPC became effective. I also contacted a doctor at Mental Health Connections (MHC), who advised me to get Mark to Dallas Parkland Intensive Care Unit emergency room. If Mark needed further help, perhaps an advocacy group from MHC would have been able to help.

Lewisville Police Department called to tell me they had Mark in custody. The police and Curt drove Mark to have a mental evaluation and review by Denton County MHMR. After the assessment, Curt drove Mark to Parkland Hospital.

Mark and Curt were not at Parkland ER when I went to meet them. Instead, I located them at St. Paul Hospital, where Mark had voluntarily admitted himself into the Psychiatric Intensive Care Unit. Once admitted, he could not be transferred from one emergency room to another, so Mark would stay at St. Paul's and be treated by their doctor.

The next day, September 29, 1994, the doctor told me that Mark appeared to be catatonic bipolar. He had rhythmic movements of bending and straightening his knees–about 50 times per minute. The doctor initially put Mark on Haldol, but after hearing that he had not done well on this medicine in the past, took him off. A meeting was planned to meet with the doctor the following week when I would take copies of Mark's medical history to him.

Friday morning, Mark had been moved to an open, less-restrictive psychiatric unit. The doctor asked about my understanding of rapid cycling and for permission to prescribe Depakote. He told me about the family meetings on Wednesday nights and said that if Mark becomes discouraged, ask him to "Please stay." He offered that Mark was a little different from other patients he had seen, and he would like to see if they could establish a rapport so he could work with him.

Later that morning, Mark called me to say that he was doing fine. The medications he was prescribed were:

Benztropine (equivalent to Cogentin) Treats movement disorders due to antipsychotics
Risperidone (equivalent to Risperdal) Treats bipolar disorder
Fluoxetine (equivalent to Prozac) Treats depressive disorder, obsessive-compulsive disorder
Divalproex (equivalent to Depakote) Treats seizures, bipolar disorder
PRN (as needed) Drugs:
Haloperidol (equivalent to Haldol) Treats agitation
Lorazepam (equivalent to Ativan) Treats agitation

On October 27th, a St. Paul caseworker called. Mark had spoken with the manager at Phoenix House. The next step was to make an appointment at MHMR. The caseworker said that MHMR was resistant to persons with a private doctor, but they could not legally turn anyone down. MHMR doctor would see Mark once per year, and MHMR would assist with medicine and housing costs.

Upon discharge on Tuesday, November 8, 1994, Mark moved into Ann Arbor House (RMI) in Dallas, where he shared a room with another resident. It was $900 per month; rent took all of Mark's Social Security check plus over $300. On Saturday, I picked up Mark so he could spend the weekend with Martin and me at home and have a change of scenery.

Tuesday, November 15th, Mark was interviewed by the manager of Phoenix House, who took an application to the Board for approval. If Mark was approved, he would move into Phoenix House, interview for jobs, acquire employment, and add stability to his life.

By Thursday, Mark called me feeling scared and had the urge to run in front of a car. He wanted to die. He said he had been watching about death on television and began thinking of his Grandma and Grandpa. I called the manager at Phoenix House. He said Mark's case would come up the following week.

Friday, Mark called again, saying he "felt all weird," and was starting to rock again (bending and straightening his knees rhythmically). When I asked him if he could control it, he said he guessed he could; I told him that I would pick him up after work, and he could plan to spend the weekend with us.

Mark and I had telephone contact nearly every night. He said he was afraid to walk in the neighborhood, which I thought was unsafe anyway. One of the attendants told me that Mark was spending far too much time in bed, sleeping most of the day. We attended a birthday party for Martin and Zach at Lynn's house on Sunday, and Mark slept part of the day. He seemed tired and distant.

Thanksgiving Day, I visited Mark at Ann Arbor House (AAH). The mother of one of the residents and the owner were there, and we all played a game called "Name Burst." Everyone appeared to be having a good time. After dinner, we drove to my sister's for Thanksgiving supper, and Mark spent the weekend with us.

On Saturday, Mark, his grandmother, and I went shopping and ran errands. Mark always felt very close to his grandma, so it was nice spending time with them.

The following Monday, the manager of Phoenix House said that Mark was approved and could move in immediately. I was glad because

Mark seemed to be very unhappy at AAH. He was assigned a bed at Gaston Road on Wednesday. The cost for this facility was 30% of Mark's Social Security check. Move-in day would be November 30, 1994.

When I notified the owner of AAH that Mark would be moving, he said to beware of theft at Phoenix House and suggested that Mark get a footlocker with a lock for his belongings. He also noted that Mark may encounter violence there, but if Mark returned to AAH, he might be able to get a job at a carpet company warehouse. I wondered why he didn't try to help Mark get employment earlier.

On Wednesday, Mark moved into Phoenix House. The manager was very helpful, checking Mark in and giving us a tour of the facility. He familiarized Mark with the rules and on Friday, accompanied him to his doctor's appointment at Routh Street Clinic.

I drove Mark to his appointment with Dr. S. the following week. Lynn asked me to submit a list of concerns she had about her brother to the doctor.

- "Why does Mark have to be so heavily medicated–so much that he cannot function throughout an entire day? It doesn't seem like he is even living, but simply existing."
- "What did you see in Mark early on that led you to believe that Mark was different than other patients he has seen? (i.e., not wanting Mark to get "lost" in the system, and the doctor taking a special interest in him.) And how are you acting on those beliefs?
- "We have seen Mark function normally on a day-to-day basis and know that he can. Why does it seem to take longer after each "cycle" to get him stabilized?"

I, too, expressed concern to Dr. S. that Mark seemed "robot-like" in his movements and that he was sleeping a good deal of the time.

Dr. S. addressed Lynn's and my concerns. He could see that Mark had considerable potential when his bipolar disorder was treated with the proper combination of medication and therapy. He explained the progression of bipolar disorder.

After I visited with Mark and Dr. S., the remainder of the appointment was a private consultation between the two of them. After the meeting, I asked Mark if he cared to share their conversation with me. He said that Dr. S did most of the talking, and that he barely participated in the session.

On Sunday, Mark, his grandmother, and I drove to visit an acquaintance of Mark's (B) with whom he had formed a friendship while they were in St. Paul Hospital. Since Mark seemed so quiet recently, I thought perhaps B could cheer him up. We visited for a couple of hours, during which time we played dominos and chatted. Mark seemed interested in the game but did not contribute to the conversation.

During that week, Mark had an employment opportunity doing janitorial work through Phoenix House. When I saw him the following weekend, he said that he couldn't work because he felt very uncomfortable taking the bus to his job. I told him that it was only temporary, and eventually, he would be able to drive his truck to work. I told him to hang in there and try.

Monday, Mark called and said he thought he needed to go back into the hospital and that he was asked to move out of Phoenix House. I told him he needed to call Dr. S. and tell him. When I asked him why he was asked to move out, he said he couldn't work. Vacuuming for 4 to 5 hours straight caused him to become hot, and perspiration would run into his eyes. I tried to convince him that the janitorial job was temporary and suggested he use a headband to help with the sweating. We also discussed the work requirement for living at Phoenix House.

During that week, Mark placed two calls to Dr. S., but neither was returned.

Mark planned to spend the Christmas holiday weekend with us.

He called early Saturday morning and asked when I would pick him up. I sensed that he was feeling lonely, so picked him up right away. Mark was extremely quiet and spoke only when asked a question. His answer was usually, "I don't know."

We were invited to Mark's cousin Denise's for supper on Christmas Eve. Mark was very quiet throughout the evening. Denise gave Mark a gift and, after the party, Mark almost took the wrong package, because he couldn't distinguish which was his.

Christmas morning, Mark revealed that he was very unhappy. He said he felt withdrawn and panicky. We discussed his current situation and possible solutions. He wrote the following:

Situation: Daily Boredom.
Solutions/Options:
> *Get out of the house.*
> *Walk to stores and window shop.*
> *Volunteer to work at radio station.*
> *Spend time in the kitchen and learn to cook.*
> *Find out if he could use his truck.*
> *Ask about a recycling job.*

Christmas dinner was at Lynn's. Mark participated in a card game, then he stayed by himself most of the time and watched television or slept in a chair. When he tried to operate his nephew's new yo-yo, I noticed his coordination was significantly diminished.

The day after Christmas, Mark, his grandma, and I went to exchange his eyeglasses. While in the shopping mall, I asked several times, "Mark, how do you feel?" He answered with, "Uncomfortable." "Strange." "A little scared." He was trying sooo hard to keep it together.

That afternoon, Grandma and I drove Mark back to Phoenix House. After we dropped him off, he sat on the front steps smoking a cigarette. As we drove away, I felt that familiar feeling of overwhelming sadness. Mark looked so sad and alone. That would be the last time I would see Mark physically whole.

The next day, Tuesday, December 27, 1994, at 3 o'clock in the afternoon, I received a call from the executive director of Phoenix House. She told me that Mark had been found lying unconscious on the ground behind Phoenix House. He had apparently attempted suicide. He was rushed by ambulance to Parkland Hospital, where Lynn and I arrived just as they were wheeling Mark out of the emergency room into surgery.

CHAPTER 7

Beginning of Hospital and Nursing Home Nightmares

December 27, 1994–February 27, 1996

MARK HAD CUT his left wrist and jumped from a second-floor balcony at Phoenix House. He wasn't breathing when the ambulance arrived, so the paramedics performed a tracheotomy. At Parkland Hospital, CT scans and X-rays revealed a severe head injury, a compression fracture in his spine, and fractures in his left leg and right wrist. Brain surgery came first: a clot and a small amount of brain tissue were removed to save Mark's life. Ten days later, bone from Mark's hip and a plate and screws were placed in his left femur. His right wrist was stabilized with a splint. On January 16, 1995, Mark was moved from the Surgical Intensive Care Unit (SICU) to a private room. While there, the hinge on his leg cast was pressing on the outside of his leg, and his position had not been changed for over six hours. Three days later, he was returned to SICU; his blood pressure had dropped to 60/palpable. He had become septic–a deadly infection was raging through his body. After five days in SICU, Mark was returned to a room on the second floor. His fever and infection persisted even though Mark was on the strongest and highest safe dosage of antibiotics (Amikacin and Timentin).

We had a glimmer of hope on Saturday, February 11th, when Mark moved his hands and attempted to move his arms; the next day, he moved his legs. Mark could not be discharged on his scheduled date, February 17th, due to his ongoing fever. The discharge was re-scheduled for Monday, February 20th. That day, Mark raised his shoulders off the bed. He had a pained expression on his face and a tear in his left eye.

Options for Mark's move to a rehabilitation facility included Baylor Rehab, Parkland Rehab, and Health South Rehab. Parkland's occupational and physical therapists were assessing Mark. He would be discharged when he was free from fever for 36 hours.

By March 10th, Mark was still at Parkland. The contrast between the excellent care Mark received in the trauma unit and the very substandard care in other parts of the hospital was glaring. I presented the nurse the following list of my observations that depicted the improper care that Mark had been receiving:

1) On March 10th, a registered nurse flushed Mark's bladder catheter with tap water instead of sterile water.
2) The contents from Mark's feeding tube was pooling in his bed instead of going into his stomach tube.
3) When moved from the intensive care unit (ICU) to Floor 2 East, Mark's temperature increased, and he was perspiring profusely. Even though the doctor had ordered a cooling blanket, it was not in use. (Three days later, Mark was returned to ICU with his blood pressure at 60/0.)
4) He lay in the same position well over the time limit for required turning.
5) The toilet in the bathroom was unflushed, and there was urine in the sink.

6) Mark's cooling blanket was heating instead of cooling, because the temperature was set too high.

7) Because it was so filthy, I mopped the entire room several times.

8) The staff dropped items (including sterile items) on the floor, picked them up, and used them as though they were uncontaminated.

9) Body alignment would go unnoticed. I would find that Mark had slid down and was curled up at the foot of his bed.

10) SCDs (sequential compression devices) were not on his legs. I located them on the floor under the bed.

11) Compression hose (TED stockings) were not used consistently.

12) Staff members were unaware that Mark's right wrist was broken; his wrist splint was lost.

13) Mark developed a large sore on his right heel from his orthopedic "space boot."

14) Mark's ears were red and bleeding. When he was turned, no attention was paid to his ears, which were folded over and lacking circulation.

15) Many times when I visited him, Mark's diaper was unchanged, and he was lying in feces.

16) I observed sterile IV paraphernalia dropped on the floor, picked up, and used as though it was uncontaminated.

17) I observed the respiratory therapist place the Yankauer Tube used to suction Mark's trachea under his arm during a supposedly sterile procedure.

18) When Mark was turned, the staff did not use care, and his nose was smashed painfully against the side rail of the bed.

Early Monday morning, March 13th, Mark was transferred by ambulance to HealthSouth/Dallas Rehabilitation Institute (DRI). They were unprepared for Mark's arrival; there was no bed available, and several members of the staff told me they did not even know that Mark was going to be admitted. Mark lay on the ambulance gurney for several hours until a bed was moved into a semi-private room for him. He had not had his morning tube feeding, and I reminded the staff several times that Mark had no nourishment all day. Transfer orders were unclear as to the time Mark's feedings were due. I was promised that a tube feeding would be ordered from the pharmacy, but Mark didn't receive his tube feeding until 6:00 p.m.

I visited Mark every day, and every day I found that he received inferior care. As early as the next day, when the nurse bathed Mark, she did not see the decubitus on his right heel, even though it was oozing through his TED hose (compression stocking). She said she "thought it was on his left heel." Why didn't she see it when she bathed Mark? No oral care had been given, so I brushed Mark's teeth and cleaned his mouth. He still had unpleasant body odor, even though he had been bathed. When we put Mark back into bed, we discovered he had had a bowel movement. When I told his nurse, she left, saying that she had to see another patient and did not return. The respiratory therapist recruited another staff member to help, so she and I cleaned Mark.

Among the things that were overlooked was Mark's tube feeding that had been scheduled at 2:00 p.m. Before I returned to work, I requested that Mark's feeding time be changed to a different shift. The very next day, his feeding had been missed, and I had to remind the nurses about it. Mark's nurse told me that Mark's 2 o'clock tube feeding had been given early. However, when she checked his chart, she learned it had been missed.

I also reminded them to bathe him more thoroughly. When I left at 2:30 p.m., Mark had not been seated in a chair, as was written on his bulletin board instructions. Caretakers seemed unaware of Mark's capabilities. I reminded them to ask "Yes/No" questions, as Mark would nod a reply if he was asked.

Several days later, I noticed that Mark's condom catheter had fallen off, so I opted to offer him a urinal rather than put another catheter in place. Later that day, he was able to urinate into the urinal. I asked the staff to offer him the urinal and bedpan to eliminate frequent bed changing and many dirty linens. Mark's nurse suggested that a bowel program be implemented.

The staff would talk about Mark while delivering care. I asked them to speak *to* Mark instead of speaking *about* him. The speech therapist had promised to provide Mark with a tracheotomy cap to make it easier for him to speak but did not deliver. At one time, Mark was able to straighten the fingers on his right hand–later, they flexed when he straightened his wrist. I wondered if the tendons had shortened. Occupational and physical therapists promised to arrange for a splint. The goals were to have Mark up at 10:00 a.m. and then do his therapies. All of these issues were addressed at Mark's Family Conference on March 21, 1995.

The following issues were presented to the staff at Mark's next Family Conference on April 4, 1995:

> 3/25/95 Lynn, Mark's sister, visited Mark's 11:00 a.m. physical therapy (PT) session. Mark's clothing and back were soaked from where the feeding tube had leaked. He was sent to PT with soaked clothing. Lynn asked that Mark be cleaned and changed when she left at 12:15 p.m. *Suggestion: Be certain Mark is clean and dry before therapy. Have Mark sitting in a chair and ready to go to therapy.*

I visited Mark's afternoon PT session. When we returned at 3:30 p.m., we noticed that Mark's 2:00 p.m. feeding had not been completely delivered due to interruption for therapy. It was finally restarted at 4:00 p.m. I asked when the next dye test could be given, so Mark's tracheostomy tube could be removed. *Suggestion: Change tube feeding time from 8 a.m. and 2 p.m. to 6 a.m. and 12 p.m.*

> 3/27/95 Tube feeding times will be changed due to interference with the 2:30 PT session.

3/28/95 Asked speech therapist when she would perform the second "blue dye"/thin liquid test. It had previously been scheduled for Friday, March 24, 1995.

3/30/95 Mark was still in bed at 2:20 p.m. His feeding tube had leaked, so he needed a change of clothing. The therapist arrived to pick up Mark, and by the time Mark was changed, there was not enough time to take him to the gym. PT was performed at the bedside–not as effective nor as comfortable.

The doctor removed Mark's trach tube. (Blue dye/thin liquid test still not performed.) Ordered a swallow test Monday, 4/3/95.

4/2/95 When I arrived to visit on Sunday, Mark's condom catheter was twisted so badly that, even though it was attached, urine went all over his clothing when he urinated. *Suggestion: Offer Mark a urinal every one to two hours.* Per staff, a urinal was offered to Mark twice during the night, and he used it.

4/3/95 I arrived at the gym to observe Mark's PT session. His therapist was on her way to pick up Mark from speech therapy (ST). When we arrived, the speech therapist told us that Mark did not have ST because he was still in bed. The physical therapists and I walked to Mark's room and found him sleeping in bed. The therapists had to get Mark up and wasted at least half of his thirty-minute session. *Suggestion: Have Mark sitting in a chair and ready to go to therapy.*

ST was rescheduled to 1:00 p.m. *Suggestion: Report to supervisor and find someone to help get Mark out of bed.*

At 2:20 p.m., Mark was still in bed. The physical therapist had to get Mark up to take him to PT. More therapy time missed. Progress noted: Mark turned on the sink faucet by himself. He also turned on the television and removed his wrist splint. *Suggestion: Have Mark sitting in a chair and ready to go to therapy.*

6:00 p.m. When I arrived, Mark's wrist splint was lying in the sink. The Velcro® was soaked. I dried it. The nursing assistant said Mark did not have the splint on from 4-6 p.m. (Nurse said wrist splint schedule was unclear; needed to be more detailed.) I put on the wrist splint at 6:30 p.m. with a note to remove it at 8:30 p.m. I removed a Band-Aid from decubitus on Mark's right heel. Arrangements were made for ComFeel and "space boots." I put on Mark's TED hose. *Suggestion: Always refer to check-off list of procedures to be carried out that is displayed in room.*

Questions and Issues:

Can Mark please be bathed more thoroughly? He is developing pimples on his forehead–never had a problem before. He very definitely has body odor.

When does he get his hair shampooed? I have shampooed it several times when it appeared very dirty, was oily, and smelled.

Does he qualify for a shower?

TED hose: on or off?

Can Mark have a remote so he can summon help when he needs to use the urinal or bedpan?

When will his trach be removed?

When will a swallow test be performed? (Mark tries to drink from his hands when he washes his hands in the sink.)

Mark has a bedsore (decubitus) on his left heel.

Mark's sister, Lynn, stayed involved in all of Mark's care, and she updated Mark's progress in newsletters to the family.

"Mark's level of awareness has increased immensely since he has moved to the rehabilitation center. His trach has been removed, and he is now eating pureed foods. When he builds up to more solid foods, his feeding tube will be removed. He goes to speech therapy once a day and physical/occupational therapy twice a day. One of the things Mark is currently working on is strengthening his trunk muscles by sitting (balancing). He is starting to use his voice; while it is quite difficult to understand him, the one word he has down to a "T" and can say real good if you piss him off is NO! Mark tries very hard, and I have observed several of his therapy sessions and am very proud of him.

"Dad and Ozzie visited Mark this past weekend (April 8th and 9th). The smile on Mark's face was instantaneous the moment they walked in the door. He could not take his eyes off of them. Ozzie even had Mark laughing on the second day of their visit. Although Dad and Oz could not stay long, it was worth every second they spent with Mark!

"One other note of progress on Mark is…as I was leaving one of my visits with him and kissed him on the forehead, I looked at him, and he puckered his lips and smacked me back! He is becoming more aware of the "goings-on" every day!"

Surprise! After being in rehab for less than one month, I was informed on April 4th that the subacute unit was going to close and that Mark would be moved to a different location where there would be no head injury specialists providing therapy until June. We fought hard to keep Mark at the Harry Hines location until all the therapists transferred to the Regal Row location in June. Without rehab, Mark's progress would suffer dreadfully. Since DRI was aware of Mark's status and his rehab's time frames upon admittance, we felt that they were not honoring their commitments. Mark had 60 skilled nursing days remaining from Medicare, and funding of $70,000 from the Texas Rehabilitation Commission (TRC) would take over when the skilled days were used. With less than a two-week notice, we were once again searching for a suitable facility that would accept Mark.

After researching three different nursing homes, on May 1, 1995, Mark was accepted at Brookhaven Nursing Center in Carrollton, Texas. Brookhaven Nursing Center was touted as having the largest sub-acute rehab center in the Metroplex.

By May 16th, the round of nursing home nightmares began. Lynn observed the aide feeding Mark by "shoveling in the food." The aide also gave Mark water even though he was on a thickened liquid diet to prevent choking. When Lynn called the aide to offer Mark the urinal, she responded, "Oh, does he use the urinal?" Lynn left the room to afford Mark privacy. When she returned, there was urine everywhere. The aide didn't know that Mark needed to have help placing and holding the urinal. I arrived shortly after that, and Lynn and I changed Mark's clothing and bed linens.

Mark's right heel was still in contact with the bed, even though he had a sore that needed to be kept off of the linens. These and other issues were presented to the staff member who attended Mark's care plan meeting on May 17, 1995. Other issues addressed were:

The sore on Mark's heel was not healing. Last evening the nurse said she had just bandaged his heel. When Lynn arrived, the bandage was rolled up and not covering his wound. There was discharge from the sore on the sheet.

When Lynn observed the aide feeding Mark, she noted that the aide needed to give Mark time to swallow (preferably more than once) then verify there was no gurgling by asking Mark to say, "Ah."

Mark's position in bed needed to be changed periodically. When I would arrive, Mark's chin was usually pressing against his chest. He needed a thin pillow, but when I went to the laundry area to get one, the only pillows I found were lumpy, hard, or misshapen. I asked speech therapists to encourage Mark to use his voice, since he would only nod his head in response to questions.

The day following Mark's care meeting, an aide was feeding Mark large bites, not allowing enough time for him to swallow. She had broken a slice of bread into pieces and mixed it with his pureed food. She was still giving him thin liquids, so when I pointed it out to her, the nurse delivered a thickener for the aide to thicken the remaining liquids. (The dietician needed to make sure patients were receiving the proper diet on their food trays.)

Mark's toe had become infected. The nurse dressed it with a Band-Aid, however, she did not use gloves, and her fingers and fingernails came into contact with the sterile area of the bandage.

A week later, May 24th, the aides were still unaware that Mark could use the urinal. During his meal, Mark indicated that he needed to urinate, so we interrupted his supper to offer him the urinal; he voided 450cc's (nearly a pint). The protector for Mark's sore heel was on the wrong foot, and his right heel with the decubitus was resting directly on the bed.

Mark's anxiety was beginning to surface. He became agitated and cried out often. He had a psychiatric evaluation and was prescribed psychotropic medication.

In Lynn's Family Newsletter on May 25, 1995, her update on Mark was very positive.

"As most of you are probably aware, we had to move Mark to a nursing home due to lack of funds. While you can probably imagine what life in a nursing home must be like, I have to admit I was surprised at what the therapists offer Mark. They work very hard with him (a team effort), and I feel they have taken a personal interest in him due to his age and hopeful recovery prognosis.

"Mark is tolerating his therapy sessions for longer periods of time. He can balance in a sitting position for a couple of minutes at a time and has more strength in his legs. He is working on strengthening his neck muscles for better head control.

"It is still very difficult to understand him, but at least now it is difficult versus nonexistent. Mark had a "modified barium swallow" test a few weeks ago which tells if everything in his throat area is working properly. The results showed that initially there was probably some paralysis in his vocal cords, which left his right side (vocal cords, muscles, etc.) very weak. But there was evidence of everything working now, so the speech therapist will work on strengthening the proper muscles, etc.

"Mark eats three meals a day now (by mouth), but still has a feeding tube which will be removed when they are comfortable with his continued progress. At times, he tries to feed himself. He does pretty good and always eats dessert (I think that runs in the family)!"

Mark's physical therapists contributed so much to his improvement. By June 5th, Mark was standing between the parallel bars, and his left leg fracture was healing well. He was able to bend it approximately 30 °. He had range of motion exercises for his arms. A clavicular fracture (of which I was unaware) had healed. He was getting physical, occupational, and speech therapy daily. He was still unable to speak due to muscle weakness around his epiglottis and nerve damage to his vocal cords. His daily nursing care still needed monitoring and remained a challenge.

Mark's 100 days of Medicare coverage was to end June 22, 1995, at which time he would be transferred from the certified to the skilled nursing or intermediate area and become private pay or Medicaid. Brookhaven needed to negotiate a contract with TRC for funding. A Texas Department of Health and Human Services application was completed to help with Mark's financial aid.

July 24, 1995, was Mark's last week at Brookhaven. We were very appreciative that their staff provided Mark the opportunity to progress to a point where he could begin more intensive rehabilitation. Lynn's Family Newsletter dated July 27, 1995, disclosed the best news of all:

"The funding came through this month for Mark's rehab. When funding from the Texas Rehabilitation Commission came through, Mom and I put on our boots and went to work to find the best rehab around. Once we established where that was (Baylor Rehab), our work was *definitely* cut out for us. We made phone call after phone call to everyone we could, to everyone they knew, and to everyone *they* knew. (I guess you would call that networking.) We were having a tough time, to say the least, in getting Mark accepted at Baylor. About two weeks later, I received a call from the doctor's office at Baylor. They wanted to meet with Mom and me regarding Mark's case. I thought this was great; they wouldn't possibly call us down there to tell us no. Well, I was wrong. Not only did they tell us no, but the doctor also made several statements "in her professional opinion" that were not easy to receive regarding Mark's prognosis. Well, let me tell you that Mom and I did NOT go down there to get a no, and by God, we weren't leaving until they heard us out!!!!!!!! (Or at least Mom.) You would have been proud of her; she is a real advocate. She talked until she was blue in the face, and I cried until I was blue in the face. I did contribute some thoughts and comments when I was able to speak. The outcome of this meeting was rather positive. They offered to accept Mark for a 24-hour evaluation, and if the therapists felt that Mark could make progress, then he would be admitted to their program. The next day I went to visit Mark and give him a pep talk. I told him how important it was that he try with all of his might to show the therapists what he was able to do. I also told him that based on his "performance," a decision would be made to accept him to Baylor's program, at which time he would be able to move out of the nursing home. He promised me he would do his best...and he did! Mom and I went to Baylor around 1:00 p.m.; Mark had only been there a couple of hours. We had only planned to stay long enough to give him our support and see how things were going. Mark was performing so well that we weren't able to pull ourselves away. Therapist after therapist came in, doctor after doctor came in, one after the other, with no breaks for Mark to rest. Finally, when Mark was to see the last therapist (physical therapy), he was so tired, and I asked if he could rest for just 10 minutes. She agreed, but upon her return, Mark was so tired he could hardly do anything. I told her I wished they had scheduled her first. Anyway, later that day, Mom received a phone call stating that Mark would be admitted to Baylor's program for a two-week trial period. (Boy, what is with these people? They just don't want to commit.) That's OK, we are moving in the right direction. Today, Mark will move to Baylor for his two-week stay. I know that Mom and I have done everything we possibly can to get Mark the best treatment, etc. Now, Mark has to want this for himself. I don't know what Mark wants, but I certainly hope he will take advantage of this situation.

"I believe Mom has come to accept things for what they are or where they may be going with Mark. However, I still have some pretty tough days. I don't know if I will ever accept things the way they are. I can only hope, pray, and give Mark all of the love and support I have. I don't know where I would be right now without Curt, my boys, and my mama, the rock!"

On July 6, 1995, approximately $60,000 TRC funds became available for two months of rehabilitation. TRC Liaison said that the territory included many hospitals, of which Baylor was the number one choice. Rehab charged $1,200 per day. Funds for 50 days were available.

After an intensive review of Mark's past records and with the help of both a fellow NAMI member and a noted Dallas philanthropist -who contacted the president and CEO of Baylor -Mark was admitted to Baylor for a one-day evaluation on July 20th. By July 27th, Mark was admitted for a two-week trial period. Therapy began the next day, Friday. There was no therapy on the weekend. When I visited Mark on Sunday, I found him lying on the floor. I wondered if this was going to be another nursing nightmare.

Monday morning, August 1, Mark's initial treatment team (doctors, nurses, and therapists) met and discussed Mark's goals. He was given two weeks to meet these goals. On August 2nd, Mark began his scheduled therapies from 7:30 in the morning through 1:30 in the afternoon. They included occupational (eating and grooming), physical, speech, and music therapy. On August 4th, I was told that plans were to discharge Mark on August 10, 1995.

At Mark's second conference meeting, the doctors reported that Mark was medically okay. He had fallen a second time during his short stay. The primary goal was to get his Tegretol level within a therapeutic range. His Risperidol was discontinued, and the dosage of Desaril was lowered to eliminate sedation and sleepiness in order to expand Mark's window of participation. Mark had used the urinal. At times he resisted his physical and occupational therapy and chose not to participate. He needed a wheelchair and equipment. The recommendation was to discharge Mark on August 10th.

I spoke with Mark's counselor from TRC. I told him that I thought time was wasted at Baylor; Mark was not there long enough to accomplish anything. Mark was unable to participate in much of the therapy, because the staff needed time to become familiar with his problems; he also was physically ill with a fever. I was very discouraged to learn that the decision to discharge Mark was made only two days after Mark was admitted. His counselor responded that a positive result of the stay was that Mark acquired a wheelchair. Of the options for discharge, he said that Mark would be transported to Healthcare Rehabilitation Center (HRC) in Austin, Texas, by ambulance on Monday, August 14, 1995.

Mark's transfer to HRC had to be put on hold due to an ongoing fever of 102°. Gallium nuclear scans were performed to locate the source of the infectious activity. Finally, at midnight on August 23rd, Mark's temperature was down to 96°. The source of the mysterious infection was never learned.

Thursday, August 24, 1995, Mark was transferred to Healthcare Rehabilitation Center (HRC) in Austin, Texas, via ambulance. I was in daily telephone contact with HRC staff. When I spoke with the RN on Sunday, I informed her of Mark's ability to use the urinal and toilet, and to speak if encouraged to use his voice. She asked Mark if he would speak to me on the phone, but he would not. Records showed that Mark had a temp of 101.8°.

On Tuesday, I learned that Mark's X-rays showed a disc fracture, a non-displaced fracture of the distal fibula epiphysis and media malleolus (ankle fracture), severe arthrosis (joint degeneration), and severe osteoporosis (weakened bones).

Thursday, August 31st, I received a message that Mark was having difficulty breathing, was on oxygen and pain medication, and had a broken leg, which was stabilized with a boot. I called the nurse, and she confirmed the info. Mark had had a temperature for two days as high as 102°. I asked when and how his fracture occurred, and she said it had been during the last 48 hours.

That evening a chest X-ray showed atelectasis (left side was not being aerated.) When I called the next morning (September 1st), the nurse told me that Mark had Adult Respiratory Distress Syndrome. His pulse oxygen was 56 (normal range is between 80 and 100), and his temp was 103°. At 8:30 a.m., he had been taken by ambulance to South Austin Medical Center Emergency Room. When I called the hospital an hour later, Mark was in the ICU on a respirator. He was heavily sedated and had a cooling blanket. His leg was in a cast and elevated. He had a lot of bleeding upon intubation, so the fluid suctioned from his lungs was bright red.

At 10:08 a.m., the doctor told me that Mark was in respiratory failure and would only live two hours without life support. I couldn't bear to let Mark die without seeing him one more time. I could drive to Austin in two hours, so I asked the doctor to put Mark on a ventilator, and Martin and I immediately began driving to the hospital.

Mark was diagnosed with mycoplasma pneumonia and a non-displaced fracture of the distal fibula epiphysis and medial malleolus. His white blood cell count was low. At 7:25 p.m. Mark's temp was down to 101°. Martin and I spent that night in a hotel and were at the hospital early the next day.

Mark had made progress during the night. He had been given no sedation since 2:00 a.m. and was resting on his own. He was not agitated, and the suction from his lungs was less bloody. He was receiving two units of blood and was breathing on his own. He needed less oxygen (from 60% to 50%) and less support from the ventilator. He was on two antibiotics: Cleocin and Fortaz. The cooling blanket had been turned off. The doctor said he was "still not out of the woods. His chances are good enough that we need to keep trying." Mark had made progress in the first 24 hours, which was a good sign. A bad indication would have been multiple organ failure. Mark had severe pneumonia. At 1:00 p.m. Mark's temp was 101.5°. By 5:00 p.m., Mark's vital signs were stable, and Mark squeezed the nurse's hand.

Over the next two days, Mark's condition improved considerably, and the doctor said it was okay to return to Dallas. So we returned home on September 4th.

Thursday, September 7th, Mark returned to HRC. The following Sunday, we visited him and found him much improved. His temperature was normal, and his oxygen had been reduced from 4 to 2 liters. He sat up for half an hour while we were there.

I had daily telephone contact with Mark's caretakers and was encouraged by the reports I received. His occupational, speech, and physical therapists displayed exceptional knowledge and patience.

For the next five months, Mark received intense therapy. We visited him every Saturday and noted how much he had progressed—both mentally and physically. He went from being quite aggressive and uncooperative to more cognizant and independent. On Saturday, September 23rd, Mark's sister, his nephews Zach and Casey, and I visited Mark.

Mark was happy to see everyone. He hugged Zach and Casey and gave them a lot of attention. Lynn and Mark seemed very close during the visit. We went outside for 30 minutes, went to the vending machine in the Bluebonnet building, and Mark played "Tic, Tac, Toe" with Zach and Casey.

The following week on Wednesday, September 27, 1995, I attended Mark's program planning meeting. Six of Mark's caretakers were in attendance. All reports were very encouraging. The 90-day admission would expire in late November or early December 1995. An Independent Living Program (ILP) would then need to be set up. I contacted Mark's counselor of TRC and told him that Mark was not ready for ILP. After the Counselor spoke with an official from Austin, TX, he told me that if Mark could make the necessary progress by November 15th, it would be possible to receive more funding.

By mid-October, Mark's new case manager reported that Mark had made tremendous progress. Sitting, balancing, stretching, and propelling his wheelchair were much improved. He had become kinder and more cordial; he even reached out to shake his case manager's hand.

After searching extensively for placement and funding options, on November 22nd, HRC agreed to take Mark on a charity scholarship for 30 days. Mark was aware that he had to "jump through hoops" to achieve his goals so that, contingent upon his progress, he could receive additional TRC funding for a maximum of six months. If Mark was unwilling to put forth the extra effort to progress from Bluebonnet to Mesa Unit, TRC could not carry him at that point, and the only alternative would be a nursing home. When I visited on November 11th, Mark wrote a birthday greeting for Zach and showed me how he could walk with a walker.

During December 1995, Mark demonstrated significant development in all therapies. He began walking with a 4-point cane instead of a walker, transferred with minimal assistance, went shopping in the mall with the staff, used more self-control, became more independent in feeding himself, and took the initiative to go to and return from his therapies on campus. He was offered a urinal every two hours during the night to eliminate using a condom catheter, and he remained continent for more extended periods of time. By December 13th, Mark was accepted by Mesa and would move into the post-acute care unit on December 27th.

The day before Christmas, Martin and I arrived at HRC by 10:30 a.m. After Mark opened Christmas gifts that we brought from his family, he wrote thank-you notes to the Harris's, Denny and Marilyn, and Grandma Brown on a sketch pad that Lynn sent to him. When Martin set the time on the watch that Denny and Marilyn sent to him, he told Mark, "You can go swimming with this watch, but don't go below 30 meters." Mark laughed aloud at the joke–the first time I had heard him laugh in months.

In the dining room, Mark began feeding himself. He did quite well at first but became upset when I told him to slow down with his cup of liquid. He became frustrated, left the table, and threw his cup, refusing to cooperate with the staff. I cleaned the table and floor and went into the day room. Soon after that, Mark moved closer to Martin and me and threw his new watch on the floor. He went to his room and sat facing the wall. Martin and I sat in the dayroom, checking periodically to see if Mark's mood had changed. It had not. After I left, Martin went to Mark's room to say goodbye, placed Mark's watch on the dresser, and told Mark where it was. We ended our visit at 1:30 p.m. – a sad ending to what began as a happy visit. Holidays can be depressing for people who do not have clinical depression, so I could imagine how much Mark's frustration and sadness were magnified by his depression.

Mark was moved into the Mesa Unit on December 27th, where many of the clients were teenagers. The transition was a bit rough. Mark was upset because his new caretakers weren't given enough information about properly caring for him. However, within two days, transfer methods were being taught to the staff by PT, and follow up by OT and ST was implemented. Mark seemed to like it in Mesa. He was initiating speech and asking questions.

When Lynn, Zach, Casey, and I visited the following Saturday, he hugged and hugged and hugged Zach and Casey. He played his harmonica and played catch with Zach and Casey with stuffed animals. We toured the building, then sat in the courtyard. Mark was verbalizing more–even tried singing. It was a great time.

Nearly daily telephone communication with his case manager kept me apprised of Mark's progress. At the beginning of our next visit with Mark, he seemed depressed, but his mood improved as the day progressed. Lynn had brought Mark a new stereo/cd tape player, and we arranged his desk so he could access it easily. We met Mark's new roommate, then went outside for a walk. After watching Zach and Casey play on the playground equipment, we visited Bluebonnet unit. We observed several things which could be improved in order to accelerate Mark's progress. Back in Mark's room, we listened to tapes, and Mark's mood improved so much that we stayed until 4:30 p.m.

Mark's first staff meeting of 1996 was Tuesday, January 16th. Grandma Brown and I spent Tuesday, Wednesday, and Thursday in Austin attending the staff meeting and monitoring Mark's therapy sessions at HRC. During the meeting, we learned that Mark needed a more stimulating environment to maintain his current level of functioning. If he went to a nursing home, he would deteriorate. Mentally, he was becoming aggressive, depressed, and withdrawn. Physically, Mark was continuing to progress slowly in speech, physical, and occupational therapies. Even though he was still depressed and lacked motivation much of the time, he was meeting his short-term objectives (STOs) for his additional 30-day stay. He was given an antidepressant to improve his mood and motivation.

I offered suggestions that would enable Mark to qualify for a more advanced program of independent living skills (ILS). My suggestions seemed well received.

Thursday morning, Grandma Brown and I went directly to the gym where Mark was scheduled to be in the standing frame from 9:00 until 9:45. Mark was not there, so a staff member called the Mesa unit at 9:15 a.m. to locate him. I walked to Mesa, and on the way, met a staff member taking Mark to the gym. Even though it was cold that morning, Mark was not wearing a jacket. I gave him mine and proceeded to Mesa. Mark's physical therapist was still sitting in the unit. When I reminded him that Mark was to be in the standing frame, he immediately went to the gym. I was not happy that Mark was missing his scheduled therapy, so the program director called a 9:45 a.m. meeting with the therapists. She addressed the behavioral, occupational, speech, and physical therapists not arriving on time for scheduled therapies and assigned specific duties to them.

By the end of January, the search for a facility for Mark was in full swing. There was a concern that Mark would not exhibit the mobility he needed to get into a group home. If Mark could not meet the criteria for in-patient hospitalization, the Texas Rehabilitation Commission (TRC) would not pay for a group home. If Mark improved and qualified to go into a group home, he could stay at Healthcare Rehabilitation Center (HRC.) If he did not improve, he would be discharged into a nursing home.

February presented a variety of challenges. Mark's eyeglasses were lost, his left toe was broken (a patient ran into Mark in the PT room), and Mark was having difficulty adapting to his leg braces. TRC had asked his counselor to freeze funding, so the counselor and I called several facilities to inquire about funding, therapy availability, and qualifications. I requested that Mark's eating program be accelerated toward the removal of his stomach tube. (Many facilities would deny admission based upon having a feeding tube.)

These and other issues were addressed at the February 13th staff meeting. Slight improvements had been made, but not the expected significant changes Mark needed to meet the necessary goals to stay at

HRC. He needed to become more independent with transfers and be able to self-motivate. He had participated well in group activities–playing his harmonica more and articulating better. His case manager asked for a recommendation to remove Mark's g-tube. Ultimately, the treatment team proposed that Mark be discharged at the end of February, as he would not benefit sufficiently to justify three more months of treatment to exhaust his funding. It was felt that funding should be reserved for long-term individual care and the treatment of regression that may occur in the future at other facilities. Also, if Mark improved sufficiently for a more intensive rehabilitation effort, he could be readmitted for another trial.

Mark was discharged from HRC on Tuesday, February 27, 1996–six months after he had been admitted. He had been accepted at Pecan Hill Ranch in Nevada, Texas, to continue his rehabilitation. Lynn, Zach, Casey, and I drove to HRC the Saturday before and packed Mark's belongings to take to Dallas to prepare for his move.

Tuesday morning, Martin and I arrived at the Austin Airport, where HRC staff picked us up. We drove to HRC and packed up Mark's remaining items. We spoke with his therapists and obtained instructions for his future caretakers. We said our "thank yous" and "goodbyes" to the people who had become a vital part of our lives over the previous six months. "Thank you" barely seemed adequate for the people who were so dedicated, caring, and committed to Mark. By 1:30 p.m., Mark, Martin, and I were on a flight to Dallas and on a new quest for more rehabilitation.

CHAPTER 8

Pecan Hill Ranch
February 27, 1996–January 22, 1999

SETTING UP FUNDING for Mark's stay at Pecan Hill Ranch was an extensive process. We worked with the Texas Rehabilitation Commission (TRC), Medicare, Comprehensive Rehabilitation Services (CRS), and Vocational Rehab (VR). The initial two-week evaluation cost was $4,200. TRC paid $2,200.00, and $2,000.00 was produced by Mark's Social Security. Mark had to apply to the Texas Department of Human Services (TDHS) for Supplemental Security Income (SSI) and set up an account with the pharmacy for his meds, which would be billed at the same rate as Medicaid.

Dr. J, the Executive Director of PHR, put my mind at ease regarding Mark's potential. Mark told her that he was happy at PHR. He was feeding himself, participating in his therapies, and showed lots of promise. I met with Mark's therapists to familiarize them with his capabilities and discuss his goals.

Cousin Joel visited Mark on March 6th. During Joel's visit, Mark was smiling, played his harmonica, and seemed less depressed.

The first staff meeting for Mark was on March 18th. All therapists, program managers, nurses, and doctors discussed short-term and long-term goals, which programs and therapies had been implemented, and how much progress Mark had made. He was adjusting well to his new surroundings, and the staff was becoming familiar with his capabilities. Within two months of Mark's admission, he was walking using the parallel bars and a walker and was able to eat a general diet. The staff welcomed my questions and telephone calls and allowed me to be an integral part of Mark's recovery. PHR was the first facility that provided me with formal typewritten reports of each evaluation and staffing meeting.

When I visited Mark at PHR the weekend of Saturday, April 6th, I noticed immediately that he was in severe pain. He was sweating profusely, and when he tried to turn in bed, he winced with pain. When I pointed out these symptoms to his caretakers, he was examined by his doctor, and X-rays were taken. On Tuesday, April 9, 1996, he was admitted to Lake Pointe Medical Center in Rowlett, Texas. The next day, he underwent surgery to replace the ball in his hip.

Many questions ran through my thoughts. What happened? How did Mark sustain a hip fracture? Why didn't his caretakers recognize that he was in distress? Did he fall, or was he dropped? It was later determined that Mark may have had a seizure that was severe enough to fracture his osteoporotic bones.

The second week Mark was in the hospital, he had his g-tube removed. He was discharged from the hospital on April 24th.

Although the setback due to Mark's hip fracture slowed his progress, his therapists continued to help him improve over the following months.

Educating the Certified Nurse Assistants (CNAs) proved to be a challenge. They were very compassionate and tried their very best to care for Mark. However, residents were allowed to defecate in the shower instead of on the toilet. This not only produced an offensive odor but clogged the drain. That issue was resolved when I explained that the smaller drain could not accommodate anything but water.

Managing Mark's medication seemed to be an ongoing concern. Miscalculations in dosage led to a shortage, so I had to communicate with the DCMHMR clinic and pharmacist to ensure Mark wouldn't run out. I sometimes had to leave work to pick up his prescriptions. The staff agreed to notify me when the drugs were nearing the end of the prescription so I could take the bottles to the clinic. Over the next few months, medication management improved.

Mark's left knee and hip healed, and he received a new motorized wheelchair. Because the double vision from his head injury persisted, he also got new eyeglasses. He was able to feed himself and perform basic grooming tasks. Still, two significant problems existed: his inability to communicate effectively and chronic, severe constipation.

Mark satisfactorily completed his CRS (Comprehensive Rehabilitation Services) program under Texas Rehabilitation Commission sponsorship, and it ended August 31, 1996. PHR Case Management continued to internally manage Mark's case and obtained certification from the Medicare CORF (Comprehensive Outpatient Rehabilitation Facility) program. After an initial payment of $5,000, PHR would use Mark's monthly SS check for him to continue to live there.

In mid-September, Mark was hospitalized overnight for a fecal impaction. The next night, Mark was rushed back to the hospital and readmitted due to profuse sweating, high fever, tachycardia, and anal pain. Mark's colon was stretched due to his inability to push, and his rectal vault was enlarged. After Mark's release from the hospital, I notified PHR staff that it was imperative that Mark empty his colon, or they would be faced with daily enemas. He needed to be closely monitored for daily bowel movements.

On November 29th, 10 of the 23 Pecan Hill Ranch (PHR) residents (including Mark) were moved to the sister facility, Pecan Tree Hill (PTH), in Greenville, TX. PTH would house Medicare, TRC, and Medicaid clients. However, after visiting the facility, I realized that it would be unable to meet Mark's needs. Texas Department of Health and Human Services did not recognize PHR as a long-term care facility (Type B license), requiring Mark to leave the premises. As soon as PHR was granted a Type B license (for non-ambulatory residents), Mark would move back. In the meantime, Mark would be temporarily moved to Dr. J's estate and personal property in Rockwall, TX, and he would continue to receive his therapies from PHR.

Until PHR could meet the standards and codes to operate as a rehab facility, the residents needed to be discharged home to their families, a licensed personal care home, or Dr. J's. The juggling of Mark and the residents began Friday, December 6, 1996, when they were moved to Dove Meadow in Carrollton, TX. Friday, as we were organizing the residents' clothing, we discovered that Dove Meadow was certified for only three clients, so on Sunday, December 8th, Mark and the others were moved to McRae House. Mark's medical records were transferred to Collin County MHMR, so he could receive his medication. By December 23rd, he had to be reinstated as a Dallas County resident in order for him to receive his meds from DCMHMR.

It was unfortunate that PHR was having so much difficulty with licensure. The Texas Department of Human Services (TDHS) recommended that PHR's license be revoked; an inspection revealed that PHR did not meet the requirements that some of the residents needed either a Type A facility (where they could transfer independently) or a Type B facility (where they required assistance to transfer). A formal hearing was scheduled for April 7, 1997, in Austin, TX. One other family member and I attended the hearing and testified on behalf of Dr. J. While trying to accommodate its residents, Dr. J. put forth considerable efforts to care for PHR clients—even to the point of moving them to her personal property until matters could be resolved.

The atmosphere at PHR was healing for the family as well as the patient. There was nearly one-on-one interaction with its clients by compassionate and caring staff, and PHR was conducive to Mark's return to what most of us refer to as normal, everyday living. Even I felt very content whenever I would visit Mark at PHR. It was as though all the clients were my friends. We would sit around the dining room table and eat, drink, chat, or play games. PHR's atmosphere was the opposite of that of an institutional environment, and certainly unlike that in a nursing home.

On January 5, 1997, Mark was transferred to Dr. J's. Ten days later, he suffered a seizure and was taken by ambulance to Lake Pointe Hospital. He was transferred the next day to Tri City Hospital then to Plano Specialty Hospital.

Mark spent three months at Dr. J's. He returned to PHR on April 18, 1997, and was there for nearly two more years.

By August, Mark was working hard in music therapy. In occupational therapy, he learned to fold and hang up his clothes. In physical therapy, he showed progress by having 25% more range in his left knee and improved muscle tone, range of motion, weight-bearing, and walking skills. He was able to share more in his speech therapy group, and he completed written exercises. His eye contact had improved, and he was using spelling to communicate. He wrote a letter to his grandmother, using great vocabulary. He had shown interest in exploring the computer, and by September, he had become quite proficient in its use. He also transitioned from his power wheelchair to a manual wheelchair and was standing in the frame for 55 minutes. He was using two words together–understandably.

Many appointments with eye care specialists throughout the year regarding his double vision were to no avail. A patch was provided for Mark's right eye, so he would open his often-closed left eye. In September, he met with a specialist from Washington and learned that there was no remedy for his double vision, which was caused by his head injury. Years later, he adjusted to his double vision and was able to function well regardless of it.

Early in 1998, Mark had been transferred to Home Health Care at PHR. In January, his weight had increased to over 200 pounds prompting a change to his diet. Music therapy contributed to the improvement of his fine motor skills. He was being re-evaluated for PT and continued to work with staff to improve his swallowing, speech, and comprehension. Mark was hospitalized on February 17th for several days to determine if he had a blood clot in his left leg. It presented as low risk because he had a Greenfield Filter in his lower aorta. In March, it was recommended that Mark move to Fountain Springs to access all therapies, but was unable to because the facility lacked handicap accessibility. By March 1998, he was showing significant improvement, and his doctor applied through DCMHMR for him to attend a day program through the Achievement Center of Texas (ACT).

In April, Mark's psychiatric problems began to escalate. He was unable to sleep at night, had episodes of crying, and became aggressive toward the staff. On April 8th, he was admitted to the Tri-City Geri-Psych Unit to adjust his psychotropic medication. Because he had no insurance coverage for psychiatric benefits, he was discharged the next day and returned to PHR. His psychiatric medication was increased, and other meds were updated by the PHR psychiatrist.

On Sunday, April 26th, several of Mark's relatives and I held a birthday party for Mark at PHR. Mark was drooling and so groggy we could barely rouse him even though he was sitting in his wheelchair. Since his change in medication, I had noticed that he drooled a lot. Over the next two months, Mark's medications were adjusted, and the side effects abated.

In May, Mark was discharged from Home Health.

By mid-September, Mark's physical, occupational, and speech therapies had been discontinued. It was taking a toll on his posture, physical strength, and bone density. His verbal communication and overall outlook were declining, and he grew bored at The Ranch. I visited him every weekend, and we went shopping or driving most of the time. He was always happy to see me and couldn't wait to get into the car, so he could have a change of scenery. Usually, we drove to Braum's, had lunch, and went shopping at Target. By the end of our treks, hours later, he was holding his head up, communicating well, and seemed more alert. Occasionally I would take a friend or relative with me; I think Mark was genuinely happy to have someone other than me visit him. I encouraged his friends and relatives to either visit or call.

In December, Mark was discharged from PHR due to lack of funding, but was re-admitted for re-evaluation under the Comprehensive Outpatient Rehabilitation Facility program (CORF).

On January 22, 1999, Mark's stay at Pecan Hill Ranch ended, and he began a year of "nursing home hopping."

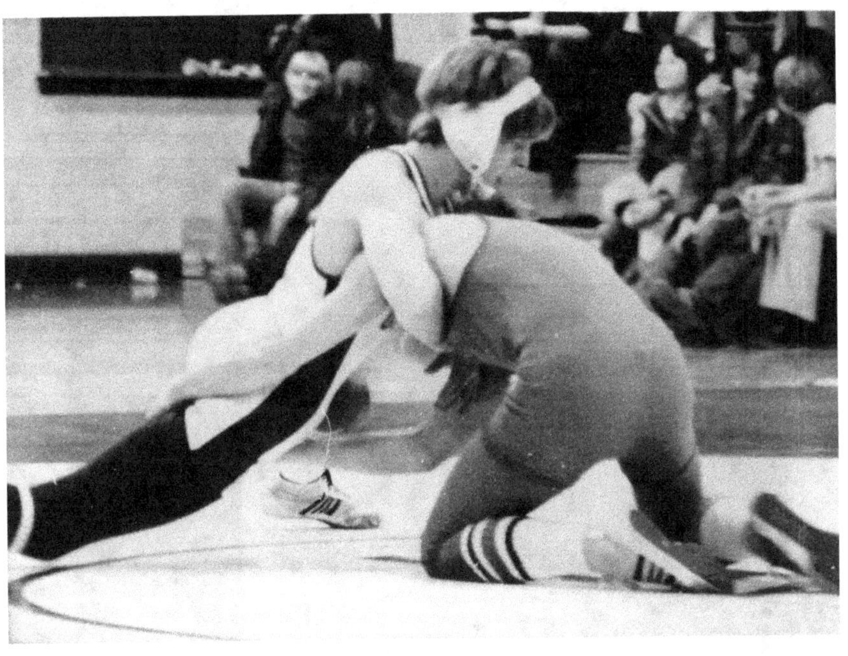

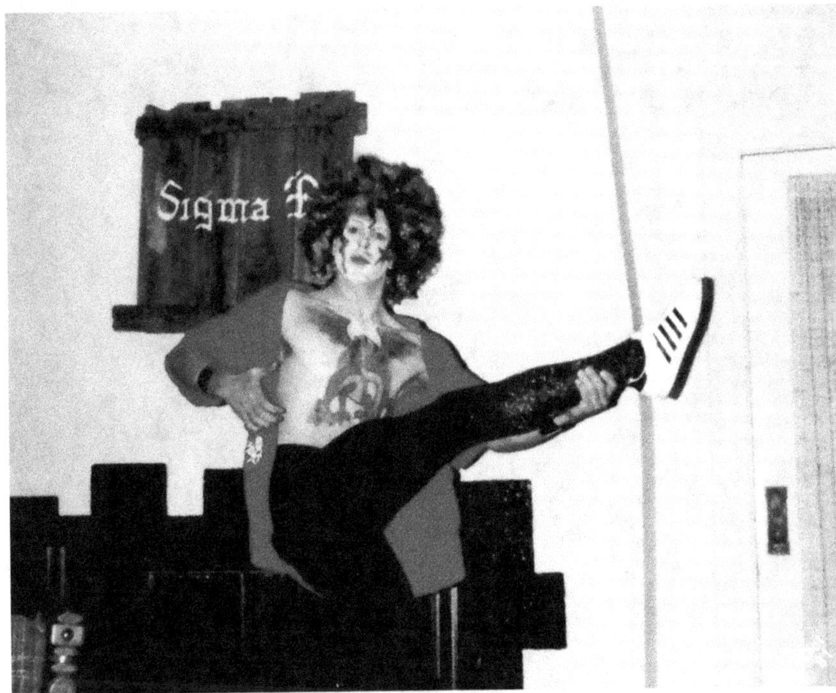
Sigma

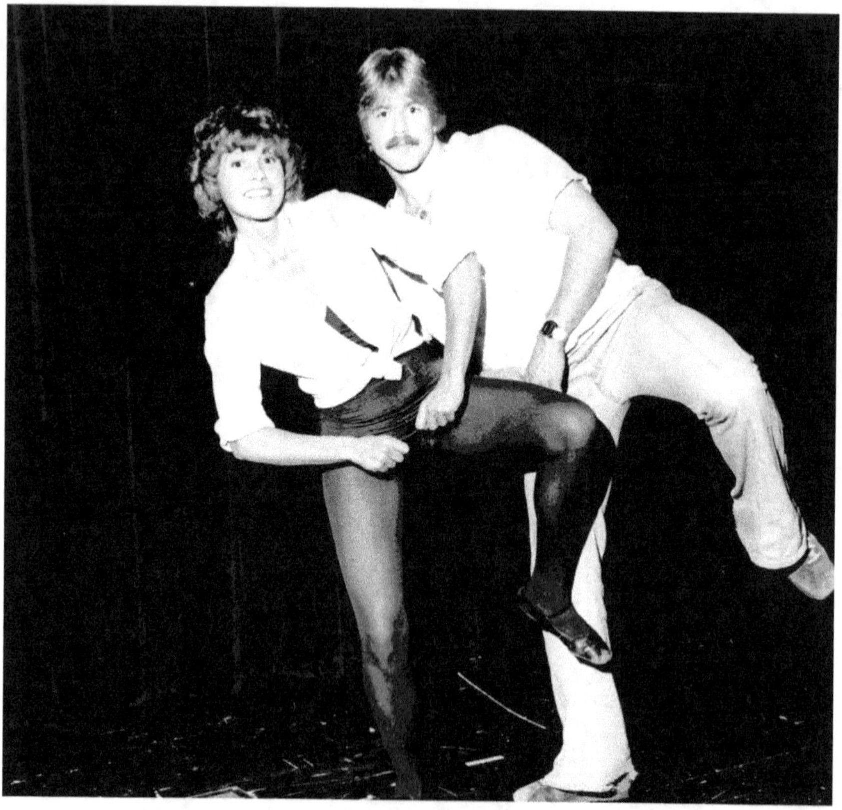

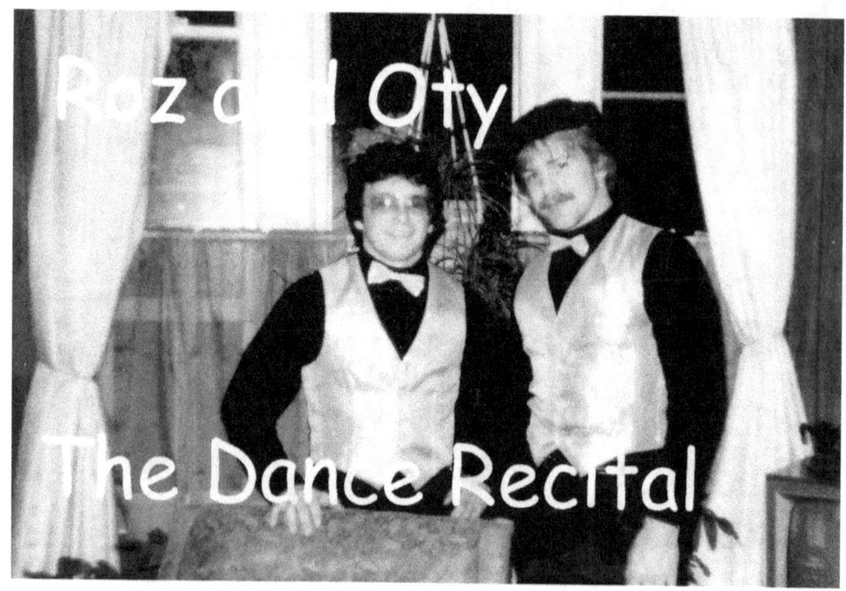
Roz and Oty
The Dance Recital

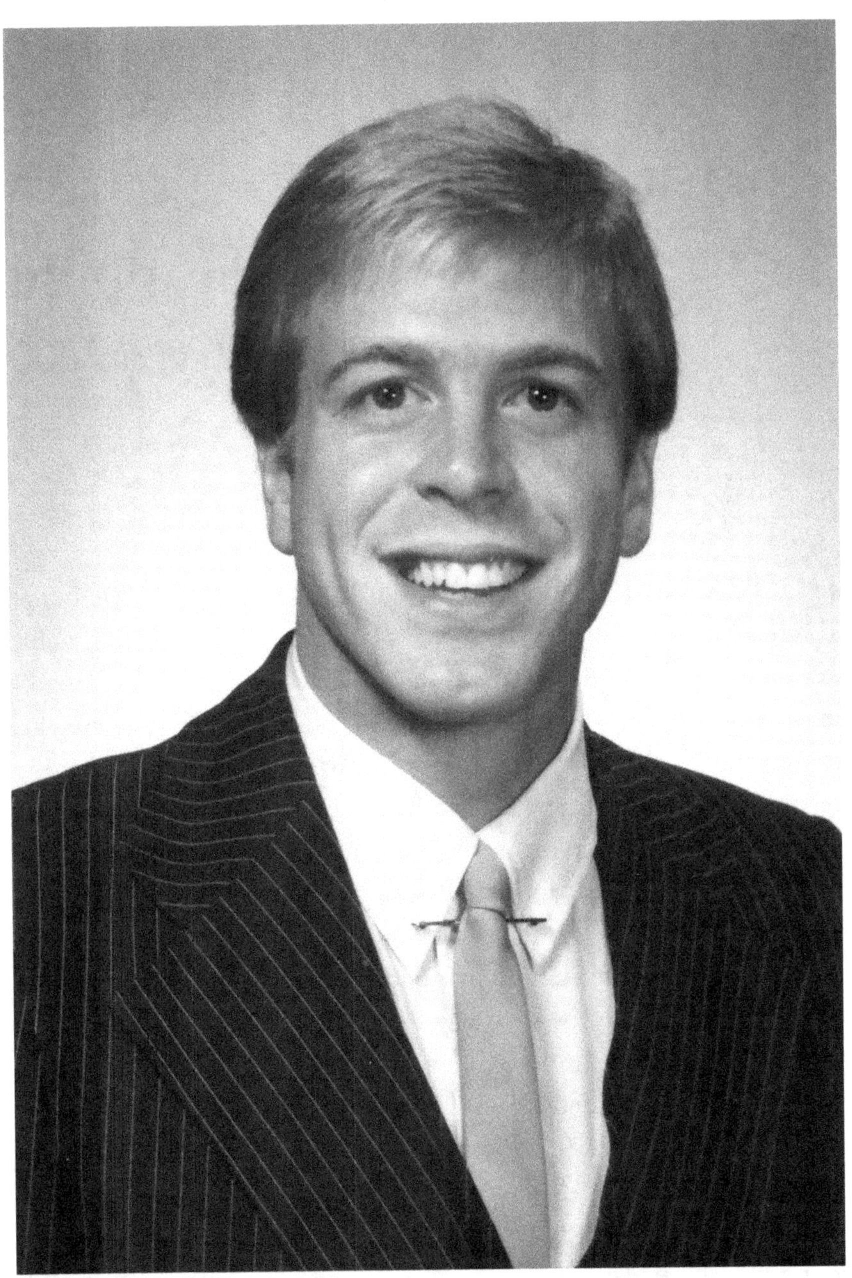

CHAPTER 9

Nursing Home Hopping
January 1999–August 2000

THE TRANSITION FROM PHR to Mesquite Tree in Mesquite, Texas, on January 22, 1999, was chaotic. Mark found relocation to his new home difficult due to communication issues, and he began striking out against the staff. He spent several days crying and punching his roommate. Neither the psychologist nor psychiatrist would return my calls. Finally, on February 1st, a psychiatrist saw Mark and gave him much-needed psychotropic medicine. Before the end of the first week, Mark had a fecal impaction that had to be removed both digitally and with enemas.

Mark was to receive his remaining two weeks of physical therapy at the Comprehensive Outpatient Rehabilitation Facility (CORF) in the Lake June facility. It was to be paid for by Medicare and Medicaid, but it was recommended that Mark receive his therapy at Community Mental Health Clinic (CMH). By February 2nd, the remaining two weeks of CORF were forfeited, and by February 9th, Mark's occupational therapy (OT) was terminated due to lack of funds. His ongoing wheelchair evaluation was discontinued "because," I was told, "the nursing home supplies chairs for the residents." The nursing home chairs were inferior and inadequate, and the quote for a new chair was $896. Eventually, after many inquiries and much effort, Mark was able to get a new customized wheelchair. He received it on February 22nd, a month after he arrived.

Following is a copy of the letter that I sent to the administrator of Mesquite Tree on March 23, 1999:

Dear Administrator,

Since my son, Mark Ostrander, moved to Mesquite Tree Nursing Center on January 22, 1999, I have made several observations regarding his care. Following are these observations, along with questions and suggestions.

1. *Observation: When I pick up Mark on the weekends, he usually has soap residue in his hair and behind his ears.*

   Suggestion: Ask staff to be sure they thoroughly rinse all shampoo and soap from Mark's hair and body when he is showered.

2. *Observation: The staff often has difficulty understanding Mark when he speaks.*

   Suggestion: Train the staff to ask Mark to speak slowly and distinctly. If they still cannot understand him, have the staff ask Mark to spell the words. If they still cannot understand, have them ask Mark to write his request on paper.

3. *Observation: When I visited Mark during mealtime, he was being fed. When I asked why the reply was that Mark makes a mess when he eats.*

   Suggestion: Please allow Mark to feed himself. Mark's fine motor skills are gradually improving, and it will certainly help for him to feed himself. When Mark visits me at home, I have him feed himself and encourage him to concentrate on using his silverware.

4. *Observation: When I picked up Mark on Saturday, he was wearing someone else's clothing. He had only one (not pair) sock in his drawer.*

   Suggestion: Because all of Mark's clothing is plainly marked with his name, is it possible for his clothing to be located?

5. *Observation: Mark's wheelchair is filthy. When I pick up Mark on the weekend, I am embarrassed to take his wheelchair in public. It is covered with food and dust.*

   Suggestion: Can you please see that the staff clean and disinfect Mark's wheelchair on a regular basis?

6. *Observation: Mark has been fitted with a new wheelchair. Since his left leg bends only slightly, the left leg rest needs to be attached. More than once, when I arrived at Mesquite Tree, I found the right leg rest attached instead.*

   Suggestion: I believe all staff members should be aware of each resident's limitations and should be trained to provide proper care.

Mark is able to use the bathroom with assistance. Can you see that he is taken to the bathroom periodically throughout the day? I feel that Mark has been allowed to just use diapers, and not enough effort is put forth to reinforce his bathroom habits.

As you know, to prevent loss of bone density, we all must bear weight at least 45 minutes every day. I would like to request that Mark use a standing frame for a few minutes each day. I realize Mark cannot have personal therapy sessions; however, is there a way that Mark can stand while others are being attended to in Physical Therapy?

Thank you in advance for your attention to my requests. I will contact you before the end of the week to discuss these issues.
Sincerely,
Colleen Nuncio
(Mark Ostrander's Mother)

Mark's stay at Mesquite Tree was brief. Apparently, the psychotropic medicines he was prescribed were not effective, and he became mentally unstable. On March 25, 1999, Mark had to be kept in his room to prevent him from hurting anyone. Later that day, his condition was escalated to urgent status, and he was accepted by Garland Community Doctors Hospital, Garland, Texas, into the Behavioral Unit until he could be stabilized. Unable to return to Mesquite Tree, it was challenging to find a nursing home that would take Mark due to his psychiatric problems. After much searching, he was admitted to The Camelot Center of Lewisville, Texas, on April 7, 1999. I visited every weekend and observed the typical nursing home problems: missed doses of medication, lack of cleanliness, wheelchair reeking of urine, broken eyeglasses, and very little therapy. By April 22nd, the Director of Nursing (DON) agreed to speak with the therapy department and have Mark re-evaluated for restorative therapy. On May 4, 1999, Mark's doctor adjusted his medication and decided to have him hospitalized for a few days to fully assess it.

The next day, May 5, 1999, he was transferred to Flow Rehabilitation Hospital in Denton, Texas. The twenty days that Mark spent there were inspiring. After being bored in nursing homes over the past months, Mark began leading the structured life he craved. He was on a time schedule, attended group sessions, and was motivated to progress. He was being treated as a human being and was recognized as a person. His eyeglasses were repaired, and an open sore on his hand was treated. The staff at Flow were to be commended. Mark left the hospital much improved.

Mark's social worker at Flow was able to find a nursing home that would accept Mark. She recommended it highly, saying that it had a high percentage of brain-injured residents and that half of them were on secured units; it had recently been remodeled and had a wonderful outdoor area. We'll see.....

Tuesday, May 25, 1999, I drove Mark to his new home at Grace Ponds Care Center in Fort Worth, TX. What a long drive! The facility was unimpressive, but we didn't have much choice, considering the lack of available places for Mark. We would make the best of it. The staff was friendly and helped me get Mark settled into his room. I told them about Mark's special bathroom, communication, and eating needs so they could more easily care for him. Over the next few weeks, while awaiting Medicaid approval for physical and restorative therapy, I requested that two of Mark's caretakers help him stand at the wall railing and walk every day to retain the skills he had learned.

After searching and searching, by November, I located a nursing home in Dallas closer to where I lived that would accept Mark. At last! I would be only minutes away from Mark! What a relief not to have to drive so far to visit. I moved Mark to IHS Forest Lane in Dallas on November 5, 1999. In mid-November, I had to spend time in Iowa for several weeks, so my husband, Martin, visited Mark while I was gone. Things were going quite well in the beginning until I received a call that Mark had struck a resident, and he was going to be discharged from IHS on November 30th. My elation turned to utter disappointment. Less than a month after his admission, he was on his way to yet another facility.

On December 1, 1999, Mark was admitted to Lancaster Health and Rehabilitation Center, in Lancaster, Texas (LHRC). Mark immediately began to gain weight. By February 2000, he had gained ten pounds. I requested that he be put on a low-calorie diet and receive only one serving of food per meal.

Mark had always been a non-smoker, but the staff allowed him to smoke when he wanted to. It was dangerous; he **received *cigarette**

burns on his finger and second degree burns on his leg. I pleaded with the staff to restrict his smoking because he had a sinus infection and cough that were being treated with antibiotics. They responded by saying that "the patient may smoke if he/she chooses to." They did, though, promise that his smoking would be supervised.

By the end of February, Mark's toe was broken as he was being transferred. After that incident, the Director of Nurses honored my request that the caretaker be retrained in proper transfer methods.

After a colonoscopy on March 1, 2000, Mark did not have a bowel movement for six days. His physician ordered laxatives, enemas, and a stool chart to record all elimination information.

Mark was finally able to get physical therapy when his orthopedic surgeon prescribed daily ambulation on the parallel bars.

From March 24, 2000, until April 14, 2000, Mark was able to take a day program at Cedars Hospital in Desoto, TX. The psychoeducational group was initially from 9 a.m.-2 p.m. five days a week from March 24th to March 31st and just three days a week from April 3rd to April 14th. Mark enjoyed meeting with the group; he was happy to have the change of scenery.

Loss of patient belongings was a regular occurrence in nursing homes, and by the end of March 2000, after I submitted the receipts, the facility replaced Mark's lost watch and some of his clothing. Loss of clothing was so commonplace that when Mark needed to leave the facility for outside appointments, I would bring clean clothing from home for him to wear off-site.

It was a long process to apply for and receive dental services for residents on Medicare and Medicaid. In March 2000, I applied for dental treatment for Mark. He received a recommendation from his doctor in April. He was able to have tooth extractions and a consultation for a partial denture in May.

The following was reported in the March 24, 2000, Care Plan Meeting.

Medical: *A second cigarette burn on Mark's leg had been treated.*

Occupational Therapy: Mark was shaving himself with his electric shaver every day.

Physical Therapy: Mark would ambulate with parallel bars daily and work on transfers.

Restorative Therapy: Mark would continue on the bars and speech therapy.

Activity Director: Art paper and an easel were ordered for Mark, and he showed a renewed interest in drawing.

Housekeeping/Maintenance: The bar in his closet was lowered so he could hang up his clothing by himself; his wheelchair seat had been washed, the brake handle was shortened, and a protective handle was added.

There had been a horrible stench in Mark's bathroom, which I reported to the administrator on April 23, 2000. The odor carried over into Mark's clothing and hair. When he rode with me, the smell even transferred to my car. The housekeeping supervisor told me that she had exhausted her resources to solve the problem. It also appeared that the toilet was leaking. A maintenance man removed the old tile in the bathroom, poured a chemical solution on the floor, and let it sit overnight. He had to repeat the process the next day, because the odor was still there. He told me that he would remove the tile he installed and try again. The issue was finally resolved when Mark's roommate was moved to a different room. It seems he had been urinating on the floor!

In addition to monthly care plan meetings, I would fax memos to LHRC to remind the staff not to neglect Mark's bowel and bladder training, inform them of therapy that had been missed, and tell them again how to manage his laundry. I felt as though I was training children who needed constant reminding of their tasks. It seemed that no matter how many times I informed the staff, I would return to see, unresolved, the exact same issues that we had repeatedly discussed.

Mark's eyeglass frames were broken in March, and Walmart would only replace them if there were no missing parts. One of the bows was missing and could not be found, so new frames were ordered on May 29th and arrived a couple of weeks later. Mark's caretaker lost Mark's eyeglasses while waiting for the frames to be delivered, so new lenses had to be ordered and didn't arrive until June 27th. As late as July 5, 2000, Mark's caretaker continued to tell me that Mark's eyeglasses had not arrived. So much time had elapsed since Mark had his eyeglasses that the optometrist personally delivered them to him.

Mark's fine motor skills were improving. He was able to use his typewriter, and he had drawn several pictures using his easel.

In early July, I received an email from Mark's Uncle Gary, who lived on the East Coast. I had kept Gary informed of Mark's progress, and he was eager to get in touch with Mark. Since his head injury, Mark's speech was difficult to understand, so I arranged for Gary to call Mark on Saturday when he would be visiting me at home. I acted as interpreter and helped Gary and Mark converse on the telephone.

Gary continued to stay in touch and offered to give Mark a computer. The computer would prove to make an enormous difference in Mark's life. Gary would provide the computer, and I would get Mark set up on email so he would finally be able to communicate with the rest of the world.

In July 2000, Mark was approved by the Texas Rehabilitation Commission (TRC) for a two-day neuro-psychological evaluation (one in DeSoto, TX, and one in Irving, TX)) and a three-day vocational assessment at the University of Texas Southwestern Medical Center (UTSWMC) in Dallas. He did exceptionally well on the tests. The person who supervised Mark's evaluation at UTSWMC said that Mark showed potential beyond just sitting in a wheelchair all day. She told me of classes where students could work on modified equipment to help improve motor skill development and suggested that TRC should be able to provide Mark with some of that equipment and arrange for him to attend classes at the Infomart. Mark had access to a computer; all he needed was a monitor and a modified keyboard. TRC granted him a Time Extension to Determine Eligibility for other institutions or special living arrangements, including group homes.

Regardless of the many undesirable living conditions, Mark continued to make progress and looked forward to living independently.

Following is a letter I wrote to the administrator of LHRC regarding observations I had made during July and suggestions to alleviate or improve Mark's circumstances.

July 31, 2000
Administrator
Lancaster Health & Rehabilitation Center

Dear __,
The good news is:

Today, Mark is in the third phase of his Texas Rehabilitation Commission (TRC) evaluation. His two prior visits (one in DeSoto and one in Irving) went well, and today is the first day of a three-day evaluation at the University of Texas Southwestern Medical Center (UTSMC). I'm sure Mark's positive evaluations will help portray the Lancaster Health & Rehabilitation Center as a stepping-stone for brain-injured patients.

After Mark's evaluation, if he should need to attend classes, I have already contacted DART (Dallas Area Rapid Transit) and asked them for an application for Mark to ride the Paratransit services. If you have any information regarding DART, I would be most interested to hear it.

May I suggest a couple of ways to facilitate getting the patients to their appointments on time?

1) As soon as the appointments are made, enter them on the patient's chart to alert the staff.
2) Alert the staff the night before the appointment.
3) Have a list of items to be completed, e.g., shower, shave, teeth brushed, etc. (Unfortunately, I have had to perform several of these items myself on several occasions.) Mark has two more days of testing to go, and it would be nice if he could be ready when we are there to pick him up.

The left bow of Mark's eyeglasses has been broken for over a week. It was very uncomfortable for him to be without the bow during his testing last Tuesday. I fully expected Mark to have his glasses for the testing today, but he was without them. Accurate testing is impeded without his eyeglasses.

I know it is impossible for you to be aware of everything that occurs at Lancaster Health & Rehabilitation Center. For your benefit, I would like to provide you with several negative observations I made during July. The observations are followed by suggestions to help alleviate or improve the situations.

On Monday, 7/3/2000, when I came to pick up Mark for a home visit, I encountered the following.

Observation: There were feces on the toilet seat in Mark's bathroom. The toilet had to be cleaned before Mark could use it.

Suggestion: Ask staff members to pay closer attention to the condition of patient rooms. Have the staff report less than desirable conditions to the appropriate personnel.

Observation: Mark was very dirty, so I took him to the shower room. The shower room was appalling. There were dirty towels, dirty clothing, and water all over the floor. This was at 2 o'clock in the afternoon. When I asked an aide to help me, she told me that this was a common occurrence; she often had to clean the shower room after the other staff members had showered their patients.

Suggestion: Train each staff member to routinely clean up after their patients each time they are finished using the shower.

Observation: Within days after the top drawer of Mark's bedside stand was repaired, the drawer came apart—and it is still broken. The repair job is far from adequate.

Suggestion: The next time the bedside stand is repaired, assign someone to follow-up. Then the problem can be resolved in a timely manner.

Observation: When the drawers of the large chest-of-drawers are opened, they do not stop but continue to move outward until they fall on the floor.

Suggestion: Place drawer stops in the chest. I would like to request that the large 4-drawer chest be replaced with two 2-drawer chests. The first two top drawers of the large chest are assigned to Mark, but since he is in a wheelchair, he is unable to see into them. It makes sense to provide him with a low chest, since he is now folding and putting away his own laundry.

7/1/2000:

Observation: When I unplugged Mark's typewriter, I discovered broken glass on the floor behind the chest of drawers. (A picture had fallen, and the glass in the frame broke.)

Suggestion: When the housekeeping staff cleans the rooms, instruct them to clean behind the furniture, in addition to the middle of the room.

Observation: When I reported a key cover missing from Mark's typewriter several weeks ago, the housekeeper told me that one had been found and turned in to the office. Will you please have someone locate the typewriter key? (I already asked the office manager, and she told me that it had not been turned in to her office.)

Suggestion: Designate where lost and found items can be placed and retrieved. Even if the finder is not familiar with the lost item(s), instruct them to turn the item(s) into the "Lost and Found" area.

Observation: When I called Mark at approximately 7:00 p.m. on Friday, I was told he was in bed already. At 10:37 p.m., Mark called me. When I asked about him being in bed so early, he replied that the nurse had sent him to bed at 6:30 p.m. because he had fallen asleep in his chair in the smoking-room. When I spoke with the morning nurse the next day, she told me that Mark had been up all night.

Suggestion: It seems that if Mark is in bed at 6:30 p.m., he will probably not be able to sleep during the usual sleep hours. I would like to request that his nurse refrain from giving Mark these instructions. (Note: Mark was moved to a different room due to a personality conflict between him and his nurse, so he now has a different nurse.)

Observation: When I picked up Mark on July 8, 2000, his supply of psychotropic medicine, Neurontin, had been depleted, so I was unable to give him his prescribed dose throughout the day. When

I returned to LH&R that evening, his supply of Neurontin still had not been replenished. The nurse on duty called Pharmerica to have Mark's prescription refilled. I do not know how long Mark was out of medicine, but he had to be given a shot of Ativan (an anti-anxiety medication) the previous night.

Observation: On July 29, 2000, the doorknob fell off the inside of Mark's door, Room 114.

Suggestion: Have routine maintenance checks to discover loose doorknobs, broken furniture, and any other items that need repair.

Observation: Mark's wheelchair is filthy. At his Care Plan Meeting on March 24, 2000, I requested that Mark clean his own chair.

Suggestion: Provide Mark with the proper tools and supervision, and allow Mark to clean his own wheelchair. Several months ago, when I requested that it be cleaned, we got cleaning supplies from Housekeeping, and together Mark and I cleaned it.

Observation: Although I have brought numerous articles of clothing to Mark, his closet looks as bare as Mother Hubbard's cupboard. He has virtually no socks or underwear left. The new shirts and pants I have bought him are either missing or have been destroyed by the laundry (bleach stains–even change of color.) Just this morning (July 31, 2000), when I spoke to Mark's Charge Nurse, she asked me what Mark was going to wear to his TRC appointment.

Suggestion: The signs posted in Mark's room and closet, stating that he will handle his own laundry, seem to go unheeded by the staff. Perhaps a meeting to educate the staff on how to handle laundry, read labels, and return clothing to its proper owner needs to be held.

When will Mark's next care plan meeting be held? The last one was March 24, 2000. At that meeting, it was discussed that Mark would continue his restorative therapy on the parallel bars, supervised by a restorative therapist. It has been four months, and Mark reported to me that he has not been on the parallel bars. I offer these suggestions to you, hoping you can use them to provide your clients with better service, and help your staff members take greater pride in their work.

Sincerely,

Colleen Nuncio

(Mark Ostrander's Mother)

Mark's fine motor skills were improving. He was drawing and writing more.

The next care plan meeting was August 17, 2000. I had a list of ten items that needed to be discussed. The most significant were the numerous ramifications of Mark's smoking. I explained that he had become thoroughly addicted. He could not afford to smoke, as his only income was Social Security, and I asked if the facility would supply his cigarettes. His smoking was to be supervised, but the staff called to tell me they could not spend as much time supervising his smoking as he needed because he wanted to smoke two cigarettes every hour. His wheelchair had several cigarette burn holes in it.

I never received a summary of the meeting. Instead, on August 21, 2000, I received a hand-delivered certified letter addressed to Mark from LHRC, giving him a 30-day notice that he would be discharged on September 30, 2000. The reason stated was, "because you will not follow the recommended treatment, and you are endangering yourself and others with your uncontrolled temper. In addition, you and your family have unrealistic expectations with regard to the role of our nursing home in your care."

CHAPTER 10

Return of Creativity and Sense of Humor

September 2000–July 2001

BY SEPTEMBER 4, 2000, Mark had moved into Kern Manor, Pilot Point, TX. It was a long drive (over an hour), but it was very difficult to find a facility near my home that would accept Mark.

TRC extended Mark's funding to help ease his transition into society. He applied for services at REACH Resource Centers on Independent Living in Denton, Texas, near Kern Manor. He was interviewed in October and November for vocational rehab and had evaluations for computer-adaptive equipment.

Mark's medications were updated, and his physical, occupational, restorative, and speech therapies were resumed. Mark was unhappy with his mechanical soft diet (pureed like baby food), so his doctor prescribed a regular diet with cut-up meat. That made his meals much more satisfying.

Mark's computer was such a benefit to him. He communicated with me via email regularly. We purchased an acoustic guitar for him so he could reconnect with his musical skills.

Consultations were arranged with an orthopedic surgeon on November 28, 2000, to address his left foot drop. His options included stretching the Achilles tendon on his left heel or having surgery to lengthen the tendon. We chose the conservative treatment of six weeks of physical therapy to stretch the tendon and strengthen his muscles. If that wasn't successful, Mark would have surgery to lengthen his tendon. By December 15, 2000, the prescribed physical therapy had not even been initiated! The physical therapist indicated that Kern Manor did not have access to the necessary equipment for Mark's physical therapy (PT). Instead, he would be transported to Denton County Hospital for it. Coordination of Mark's hospital appointments was problematic. Lack of communication among the staff resulted in missed, canceled, and rescheduled appointments. Because of the holidays, Mark was unable to receive PT until January 5, 2001–which he got at Kern Manor. Due to the delay in PT, Mark's six-week Achilles tendon checkup had to be rescheduled for February 21, 2001.

On December 12th, Mark acquired a roommate with whom he became friends. How encouraging it was when Mark began to show an interest in others! He also regained his interest in writing poetry. Mark, with the help of the staff and other residents, created this poem:

Only One knows where the wind blows,
And where it comes to.
I love you,
I love you.

Billy wants to 'moke,
While Barry tells his jokes.
It is not for your ears to hear,
What I think about Kern Manor.

This is a nice and healthy place,
For those who need their own little private space.
We wait for Helan and Ruby and sometimes Dawn,
To help us get along.
Help us get along.

Only One knows where the wind blows,
And where it comes to.
I love you,
I love you.

The nurses are nice
And this is a nice place to live,
Just give them a chance and they will always give.

Two to ten is the best shift to work,
And being around Shawndra will always give you a perk.
Angela is so perky and neat,
Just talk to Karen-she thinks Angela's sweet.

Angela quit and that made us all sad,
Because she was one of the best we had.

Kathy is always cool and calm.
She always gets the job done,
Because she's the bomb.

Tim's always at work.
But he's not in it for money,
We know he's here to find him a honey.

Wanda's eyes are blue as the sky.
Look at her dimples,
She's such a cutie pie.

Barbara is a friend to us all.
Just look over your shoulder and give her a call.

Twila and Tim are a cute pair.
One is dark and one is fair.

Only One knows where the wind blows,
And where it comes to.
I love you,
I love you.

Jo works morning, noon, and night,
Something about this just ain't right.
Brenda works at night,
Chad knows piano, he is willing to fight.

Dan is the boss of us all,
And he is the nicest of us all.
A swell guy he is.
Tim is the coolest,
He knows how to get your mood up,
And that's the best... By the Staff and Residents of Kern Manor

Mark's sense of humor was returning, too. This email that I received from him January 5, 2001 at 7:00 pm made me smile:

Dear Martin and Mt's queen,

My cup is the 2nd best thing I like best besides my smokes, computer, and my long hair, and delete key.

Could you get with Michael, Jeff's son, to scrounge around for a hard cover dictionary and rhyming book 'hard cover', it's time to get to work.

Love, Mark

Email at 9:00pm.

Martin's queen,

I went to P.T. today. But I cheated on the standing board. I kept most of my weight on my good side. I still have a bum left leg.

Love, Mark

For another example of the return of Mark's sense of humor, here is an email that Mark sent to his Uncle Gary on January 15, 2001:

Dear Gary,

A young man by the name of Johnny was listening to his teacher when she said, "The one who answers this next question gets to go home early."

She asked, "Who said, 'I have a dream.'"

Jennifer responded quickly, with "Martin Luther King, Jr." This made Johnny angry because he knew the answer, but didn't get called on.

She said, "Ask not what your country can do for you. Angela was called, and she said, John Kennedy. By this time, Johnny was furious. He said, "I wish these bitches would keep their mouths shut." The teacher reeled from the board and asked, "Who said that?"

Johnny stood up beside his desk and said to the teacher and class, "Bill Clinton. There, may I go home early?"

I spent every Saturday with Mark. Some Saturdays we drove to his sister's house in Lewisville, Texas, and spent time with her two sons, Zach and Casey. They were an essential part of Mark's life. On Saturday, March 3, 2001, Zach and his friend went to Kern Manor with Grandma Brown and me. As a school assignment, they would clean and organize Mark's room. We were there from 10:30 a.m. until 5:00 p.m. Zach documented the project in a scrapbook with pictures and writing to receive credit. What a great day!

I sent a fax to the staff on March 19, 2001, with some suggestions to help Mark gain his independence. He had gained a considerable amount of weight, and I requested a low-calorie diet. I discontinued bringing him snacks (mostly mixed nuts), and he was drinking only diet sodas. I asked them to remind him to brush his teeth regularly and shave himself instead of having the staff shave him. He needed to be encouraged to lift his head and pull his shoulders back instead of slumping. Since he slept in his clothing many nights, he needed to have clean clothing daily. The staff needed to be reminded that Mark's dirty laundry would go into his mesh bags, and would be laundered in those bags. On Saturday, when Mark's grandmother and I visited, we spent nearly two hours sorting clean socks from the laundry room, only to learn from a staff member that the socks were all tossed together and were not sorted by name. Only when they were needed were they taken from the communal batch, paired with a suitable mate, and distributed to the clients-regardless of ownership. We found only two pairs of Mark's socks-and they were no longer white, but a dingy gray, or blue, or pink, or whatever color the white clothes may have been washed with.

On March 21, 2001, Mark went to Denton Community Hospital, where he had surgery to stretch his Achilles tendon. The surgery went well. Mark was a good patient. That evening, he sent this email to his father, Dennis Ostrander:

Dear Dad,

I'm so glad we can talk like this. It makes me feel like I was stuck in a well screaming and you were there pulling me out. Today I went in for surgery to stretch my Achilles tendon. Please don't check my spelling, you know what I'm talking about anyway. Maybe someday I will walk again.

Love,

Mark

Mark's poetry was coming together again.

Don't kiss me too hard, I might wake up.
Might wake up, might wake up.
I don't even want it to be a dream,
Be a dream, be a dream.
I love you more than words can say,
I love you more than words can say, words can say.
I shouldn't have let you do it
I know it was wrong all along.
But you captured my heart,
Captured my heart.
I know when you're around,
I can smell your sweet perfume.
It's almost as if you were in my room,
In my room.
Don't let loose your sweet caress,
Or your sweet love and tenderness.
I couldn't take it,
I know I just couldn't take it.
Cupid lost an arrow,
And it fell on you and me.
Fell on you and me.

Kern Manor supplied forms to the National Heritage Insurance Company (NHIC) with incorrect information regarding Mark's Medicaid eligibility. In April, NHIC determined that licensed nursing care was not medically necessary, and Mark was denied Medicaid. We appealed the decision and petitioned the Texas Department of Human Services (TDHS) for a hearing, which was granted for May 21, 2001. In June, we received notice that the decision was reversed, and Mark's Medicaid was reinstated. Issue resolved–after three months of worry--due to one incorrect answer on an application!

April was filled with doctor appointments and post-op physical therapy. Mark was becoming proficient on his computer and continued to email and telephone me. He would watch nearby ballgames from the back of Kern Manor. One day he decided to actually go to the game and wheeled himself into the street. Fortunately, the staff discovered he was missing and rescued him before he was struck by a car. He had his cast removed near the end of the month and began additional therapy.

In May, TRC agreed to continue to pay for Mark's rehab services as long as funds were available and Mark continued to make progress towards an employment goal. He would receive counseling and guidance, and classes for basic computer skills training through June of 2003.

Every email I received from Mark filled me with hope for a promising future for him. I could see the progress he was making and sense his interest in life return. He was more aware of what was happening around him and interacted much better with others.

All good things must come to an end. On Thursday, July 5, 2001, Mark was admitted to Garland Community Hospital for psychiatric evaluation. He had hit another resident, had a confrontation with a staff member, and bruised the side of a nurse's face. When I visited him on Saturday, he was remorseful and cried. He was filthy (had not had a shower for two or three days) and had dried feces on his bottom.

His caretaker and I helped him shower and brush his teeth. We put his clothes in the laundry for the staff to launder. Mark was in a room with no handicap bars in either the bathroom or the shower. I requested a handicap room for him, which went unheeded.

I visited Mark again on Sunday and took him two packs of cigarettes with instructions for the staff to give him no more than two cigarettes every two hours. We showered him again. He had missed the toilet when defecating, so we cleaned the feces from his bottom and the toilet. Once again, I requested a handicap room for Mark. How on earth was he able to get from the wheelchair to the toilet without a handicap bar?

When I visited Mark Monday evening, he was still wearing the two gowns that we had put on him after his shower on Sunday. Both packs of cigarettes were gone; he had smoked them between 4:00 p.m. on Sunday and 7:30 p.m. on Monday. I asked the staff a second time to ration Mark's cigarettes.

On Tuesday, I asked the technician to please help Mark dress and brush his teeth and hair. He said he would request a physical therapy order for Mark, which was granted on Wednesday. On Thursday, he had his first PT session. The doctor ordered Celexa for Mark's mood swings, though he had exhibited no aggressive behavior since he was admitted.

Mark's social worker let me know that Kern Manor (KM) would not take Mark back. If they did, the resident's family would press charges against both Mark and KM. We began exploring options of nursing homes that would accept Mark after his discharge on Tuesday, July 17th, but found none. The doctor changed the discharge order to Wednesday, since Mark had no place to go, even though he did not meet the criteria to remain in the hospital. Homeless shelters seemed to be the only alternative. Then, at last! After being denied by nearly a dozen facilities, Mark was accepted by Silver Leaves in Garland, Texas.

CHAPTER 11

A Year of Adapting
July 2001-July 2002

AFTER SPENDING THREE weeks in the Garland Community Hospital, Mark was admitted to Silver Leaves Nursing and Rehabilitation Center (SL) in Garland, Texas, on Friday, July 20, 2001. The only room available to him had a narrow bathroom door that he could not navigate with his wheelchair. Until he could be moved into a room with a wider bathroom door, Mark would use the shower room bathroom, just a few feet down the hall. After supper, I helped Mark use the bathroom, take a shower, and brush his teeth. I gave Mark's cigarettes to the nurse and asked her to give him no more than two cigarettes every two hours.

On Saturday, Martin and I hooked up Mark's computer. His doctor wrote orders for physical, occupational, and speech therapy.

Sunday, I picked up Mark and took him to our condo. We had a pool party with his sister and her family. Mark was able to stand in the pool and take several steps holding onto the side.

On Monday, there were still no appropriate rooms available for Mark. In the evening, his Grandma and I visited; we toured the facility, took Mark to the smoke room, and stayed until 9:15 p.m.

Tuesday evening, Martin and I visited Mark. The nurse told us that Mark was smoking more cigarettes than allowed. Again, I asked that his cigarettes be rationed. Gradually, things were getting set up so Mark would feel comfortable in his new home. I had made arrangements for a phone line to be installed on Monday, July 30, 2001, so Mark's phone could be transferred to SL.

Mark's physical therapist spent a lot of time helping Mark with all aspects of his transferring, standing, and walking with a walker. So helpful! She explained how we could help Mark practice walking sideways in the hallway holding the hand railing. His occupational therapist encouraged Mark to use the urinal rather than the shower-room bathroom. She suggested getting Mark an electric shaver, and she would have him shave in OT. To improve his balance, she had Mark stand holding his walker with one hand and throw balls into a basket with the other.

When Grandma and I visited Mark on Thursday evening, there was an overflowing pan of water on the floor beneath the bathroom sink. I notified the nurse, soaked up the water with several pads, and turned off the water valve coming into the sink. Maintenance was to have repaired the leak the next day. When we returned on Saturday, the hot water was still leaking in the bathroom sink.

Saturday, Grandma and I picked up Mark, ate lunch at IHOP, and went shopping at K-Mart. We purchased a zippered bag and a hanging bag for him to transport personal items to the hall bathroom. When we returned on Sunday, the hot water was still leaking in the bathroom sink. The nurse said the leak would be addressed on Monday.

Mark's fine motor skills were steadily improving, and he was able to write legibly. His smoking addiction remained a problem; he wanted to smoke every 30 minutes instead of waiting for an hour between smoke breaks.

Mark had been incontinent of urine, so I asked the nurse to please ask the staff to be sure that Mark went to the bathroom in the morning as soon as he got out of bed. Incontinence could be avoided, since he knew how to use the bathroom. We discussed Mark's ongoing constipation. After not having a bowel movement for nearly a week, I asked that the doctor write an order for an enema. Success! After the enema, he had a BM in the toilet.

We included Mark in family events at every opportunity. Saturday morning, I picked him up, and we drove to Lynn's. We had a pizza lunch and returned to SL at 4:30 p.m. Sunday afternoon, we attended a birthday party for Mark's Aunt Joan at his cousin Jeff's.

Mark told me that he had been incontinent on the way to the shower Sunday morning. The staff and I decided to address the problem by asking him to use the bathroom before he went on smoke breaks. To keep track of his activities, I created the following chart where each activity was recorded and initialed either by Mark or a staff member.

Y=Yes, N=No, I=Incontinent

7/29/01-8/4/01							
Activity	Sun	Mon	Tue	Wed	Thu	Fri	Sat
Bathroom	I						
B M	N						
Br Teeth	Y						
Shave	N						
P.T.	N						
O.T.	N						
S.T.	N						
Shower	N						

8/5/01-8/11/01							
Activity	Sun	Mon	Tue	Wed	Thu	Fri	Sat
Bathroom	I						
B M	N						
Br Teeth	Y						
Shave	N						
P.T.	N						
O.T.	N						
S.T.	N						
Shower	N						

On Wednesday evening, August 8, 2001, Grandma and I visited Mark at 8 p.m. He needed to be showered, shaved, and have his teeth brushed. He had not had a bowel movement, so I gave him an ounce of Colon Cleanse (psyllium husk) in juice and water. Then I observed while he shaved with his electric shaver. Next, Mark brushed his teeth in the shower bathroom. He had a LARGE BM (observed by a staff member and me). It was so large, the toilet would not flush. I retrieved it with gloves, then helped Mark shower.

Mark told me that he had been incontinent (of urine) twice in the a.m. after breakfast. The staff member checked, and two medium BMs were charted–although Mark said he had not had a BM. (Which was accurate?) The staff member also said that Mark was never incontinent on her afternoon shift. I promised Mark that if he remained continent the next day, we would go out for a malt. The next evening, Grandma and I visited Mark. He had remained continent. After he shaved, brushed his teeth and his hair, we took him out for the promised malt. It was so nice having Mark nearer to home so I could monitor his progress more closely.

By the end of August, Mark had declined significantly, which led me to request a change or decrease in the dosage of his psychotropic medication. He had become incontinent, lost interest in his computer, and it was more difficult to understand him when he spoke. Before this, he was extremely interested in and excited about his computer. He went from staying up late at night typing poetry and corresponding with his family and friends via email to seldom accessing his email or even turning on his computer. When I visited him on the evening of August 31, 2001, he had 16 unopened messages in his email. Staff members told me that Mark spent most of his time lying in bed or smoking cigarettes in the smoke room. His progress was also declining in physical, occupational, and speech therapy. Initially, when he began PT, he was able to walk, assisted with a walker, approximately ten feet. When I observed him on August 30th, after he took three (very shaky, uncoordinated) steps, he sat down in his wheelchair. On September 4, 2001, the order came through from Mark's psychiatrist to discontinue Trazodone (50mg), decrease Depakote from 500mg to 250mg, and decrease Zyprexa from 10mg to 2.5mg. Those changes in his meds led to an improvement in all areas. He apparently had been overly medicated.

November 15, 2001, was Mark's care plan meeting. Even though I was notified only the day before, I was able to attend. I sent a memo to his social worker, telling her about the late notice. I also told her that I had called on November 14th to give them notice to have Mark ready for me to pick up by 5:30 p.m. so we could attend a 6:30 p.m. gym class. When I arrived, he had not been shaved, so I wheeled Mark to the bathroom nearest his room (shower room) only to find there were laundry barrels blocking the door and feces all over the toilet and sink. I recognized this as Mark's mess, since he had very recently had diarrhea. (Mark had been given a shower after his messy bowel movement, but the toilet was never cleaned.) I asked the staff to please clean the bathroom so Mark could use it. When we tried again to use the bathroom, it had not been cleaned properly–there still were feces on the bowl of the toilet and on the sink. Being in a hurry, we went to the next bathroom down the hall, but it was not equipped with handicap bars, and Mark was unable to use it. We returned to the shower room, and eventually, he was able to use it. Needless to say, Mark and I did not make it to our class.

When I checked Mark's laundry to determine if he had been incontinent, I could not locate any underwear in the laundry bag. The aide in the room informed me that Mark was currently not wearing underwear; since he was not wearing any before his shower, she assumed he did not wear any. (If she had asked, Mark could have shown her where to find it.)

I asked her to set up a definite schedule for Restorative Therapy and Activities of Daily Living (ADLs). It was my understanding that, because his progress was declining in all his therapies, he was to have restorative therapy every day. However, it became so inconsistent that I visited Mark during my lunch break from work so I could help him walk using the parallel bars and move from his wheelchair to a walker. I also requested that Mark be allowed to shave himself with his electric shaver (with supervision) as an ADL. Obviously, that had not occurred.

I attached a copy of the fax that I sent to Mark's doctors and to the SL Director of Nursing regarding Mark's decline in progress and request to change or decrease his medication. I let her know that since changes were made to his medication, he had shown significant improvement.

At his care plan meeting, I learned that Mark was incorrectly diagnosed with hypertension (high blood pressure). We discussed his incontinence, decline in progress, smoking, and personal hygiene. The nurse planned to schedule a urinalysis to address the incontinence and set up a bowel and bladder program. The director of physical therapy would re-evaluate Mark for eligibility to have PT. The restorative therapist would implement ADLs, including shaving and standing. The social worker agreed to refer Mark to a psychologist and to research a day program. (Ultimately, he was denied access to the day program.) Medication was adjusted to address his diarrhea.

When I picked up Mark on Thanksgiving, his partial denture

(which had three teeth) was missing. The CNA and I searched his room, the shower bathroom, and the smoking room; we could not find it. The next day I sent a memo to the DON and asked her to check with the laundry personnel in case it was accidentally put in the laundry with his bed linens. A week later, it still wasn't found, so the social worker made a dental appointment for Mark, so a new one could be made.

Mark began having restorative therapy every day. Since Mark's left leg would not extend fully, his therapist recommended the sole of his shoe be raised so he could bear more weight on it. He was taking ten steps on the parallel bars and going to the gym with me. After kickboxing class (yes, he took kickboxing in his wheelchair), we would hit a few racquetballs, then stop and pick up a hamburger on the way back to SL. We were communicating again via email. If Mark had computer questions, I would answer them via email. It was good to have Mark involved and participating in activities again. He was trying sooo hard!

By December 20, 2001, a dentist was located who would build Mark's new partial denture. Mark needed a tooth extraction, so the search began to find a dentist who would accept Medicaid. Finding medical specialists who accepted indigent patients always involved extensive searches. Very few accepted Medicare and/or Medicaid.

The year 2002 began with more time spent in the hospital. On January 7th, Mark fell. He was admitted to Doctors Hospital in Garland on January 8th, with a temp of 101.6° and a diagnosis of pneumonia. By January 10th, Mark's left leg was red, hot, and painful. He was diagnosed with deep vein thrombosis (DVT) in his left leg and was prescribed blood thinners and pain medication. His incontinence was addressed, and he was checked for infection and urine volume. It was also discovered that his bladder had become distended, and he would need to empty his bladder more often. He returned to SL January 14th. He continued to be incontinent, so I again requested that the staff continue to observe his bladder training program.

In March, Mark received notice that he would be discharged from physical therapy, which he had been receiving five days each week. Instead, he would receive restorative therapy three days per week. Speech therapy would continue, and Mark's diet would be upgraded from puree to mechanical soft. If I hadn't visited Mark as often as I did, I feel that he would have just deteriorated. I was constantly monitoring his progress and communicating with his caretakers.

Mark stayed at Silver Leaves for nearly a year. In July 2002, I moved him to IHS of the Village at Richardson, Texas, which was closer to where I lived. I could spend more time with Mark, and, hopefully, he would receive more consistent and improved care.

CHAPTER 12

Four Years of Frustration
July 2002 –September 2006

JULY 18, 2002, Mark moved to IHS of the Village at Richardson, Texas (The Village). Changing nursing homes required a lot of effort. Besides moving all his possessions, his computer needed to be connected, and his phone installed. He had to change telephone providers, so didn't get his phone connected until August 14th. I provided Mark's caretakers with information about his capabilities, his daily dental routine, bathroom schedule, and smoking guidelines.

With Mark only blocks away from where I lived, many times after work I would pick him up and drive him to our condo where I would help him hit tennis balls from his wheelchair on the tennis court. It provided him with much-needed exercise and improved his coordination.

Problems arose in August with the bathroom. The oversize potty seat hindered Mark from entering the bathroom without moving the seat away from the toilet. When he used the toilet, his urine and feces went on the floor. When Housekeeping was paged, they would not show up to clean, and although Mark needed to be taken to the bathroom, the CNAs were seldom available. August 9, 2002, Mark was moved to a different room. Hopefully, that would solve the bathroom problems.

On August 20, 2002, Mark was discharged from speech and occupational therapy. He would continue with restorative therapists, who would be trained to care for Mark.

A remarkable man volunteered to help Mark with his guitar. I met with Mark and his tutor on Friday, August 29th, and they set up times for Mark's lessons. How generous of him to give Mark this opportunity! He converted Mark's 6-string guitar to a 4-string to make it easier for Mark to grasp with his compromised hands. He also presented him with a guitar strap. The lessons were held either in the reception area or in an outside area at The Village. Mark's tutor became a significant part of Mark's life during that time.

As I continued to monitor Mark's living conditions, I realized the bed in his new room was too high for him to transfer safely to and from his wheelchair; the bed rail was in the way of his transfers, and the bed wheels did not lock securely. On September 4, 2002, I requested a different bed, and it was replaced.

Mark was still depressed and would sometimes refuse to shower. His CNA would telephone me, and I would become the mediator/negotiator. "You need to have a shower so I can pick you up on Saturday," and he would agree. He would hand the phone back to his CNA and tell her, "OK." I maintained a good rapport with his caretakers, and if Mark was being difficult, they knew they could always call me to help make their jobs go more smoothly.

Mark's best friend from college, Roz, and Roz's sister, Mindy, remained faithful friends and continued to stay in touch with Mark via mail and email for the rest of his life. Roz visited Mark at The Village in the summer of 2002 and really lifted his spirits. He stayed for several days and visited Mark every day he was in Dallas.

TRC continued to monitor Mark's progress and his needs for technology resources. On October 2, 2002, a TRC rehab engineer evaluated Mark for computer equipment. Good news! Mark qualified for upgraded equipment.

Topics covered at the Care Plan Meeting on October 29, 2002, were quite similar to the previous meeting. When the nurses gave water with meds, they dumped it into his mouth, and he would choke. I suggested that the nurses allow Mark to hold the glass while drinking to control liquid intake and avoid choking. My requests were simple: that the nursing assistants take Mark to the bathroom first thing in the morning so he would stay dry during breakfast, that housekeeping personnel use clean water when mopping to avoid sticky floors and unpleasant odors, and that speech therapists change Mark's diet to mechanical soft. The activity director had positive news and reported that Mark was actively in his wheelchair more often and was getting weekend outings with family.

In December 2002, the administrator was replaced. While Mark lived there, The Village changed administrators numerous times. Change of staff was commonplace in nursing homes. Administrators barely lasted a year.

By the New Year, Mark had been moved to room 1204. At the January 28, 2003, Care Plan Meeting, many of the previous problems had been resolved. Still remaining were Mark's bathroom issues. Mark needed to be encouraged (and allowed) to use the bathroom by himself. I asked that a second grab bar be installed in the bathroom to make it easier for him to use the toilet.

Sunday, March 9, 2003, I received the following email from Mark:

> *Mom,*
> *Sorry I tried to kill myself.*
> *Guess I could fuck up a wet dream if I had the chance.*
> *Luv,*
> *Mark*

Mark seemed to be contemplating his life actions and was aware of his suicide attempt. How do you respond to a statement like that?

I always encouraged Mark to stay positive, not regret what happened in the past, and look forward to the future. Mark would often become very depressed, and I think that he would have made a second attempt to take his life if he had the opportunity.

It wasn't uncommon for the residents' possessions to be lost, stolen, or broken in nursing homes. Mark's electric shaver was broken in March. The Village replaced it, so in order to keep it safe, it was placed in a secure area. I would retrieve it when I visited Mark and help him use it before lunch each day.

At the April 2003 Care Plan Meeting, I requested a restorative therapy (RT) evaluation because Mark had trouble maintaining his balance just to stand. It was agreed that he would begin RT on May 12th. (But it did not occur until June 11th.) Due to his weight gain of 12 pounds since January, he would have fruit instead of sandwiches for a 2:00 p.m. snack.

At the end of May, Mark received his new computer, monitor, and keyboard. His coordination and fine motor skills had improved so he could advance from a "Big Keys" keyboard to a standard keyboard. He was happy to have the new equipment and welcomed the new challenge.

Mark's roommate was outgoing, cheerful, and an excellent advocate for Mark. I looked forward to seeing him when I visited Mark. Many times I would call him, and he would tell me what was happening with Mark. One evening he and I were speaking on the telephone when the nurse gave Mark his pills. Even though Mark began choking, the nurse left the room. His roommate turned on his call light, but no one responded. So, I called the nurses station from home and told the nurse who answered that Mark was choking. She went to his room, and I again called his roommate. When he answered, I could still hear Mark coughing in the background. I asked the nurse to chart the incident and make sure that the nurse who had given Mark his pills was taught to NOT leave a patient when he/she was choking!

Mark's CNAs were less than thorough. I often wondered if they had any common sense. When I visited Mark one day in June, I noticed that his clothing and bed linens were wet, but the diaper he was wearing was dry. It appeared that he had been incontinent, but only his diaper was changed. What??!! So I changed Mark's clothing and his bedding. Then I sent an email to the supervisor asking that the staff be trained to change all wet items, not just the diaper.

The CNAs' negligence was evident in so many ways. Many times when I visited Mark on my lunch break, he was not wearing his partial denture. "Why didn't he have his teeth cleaned in the morning so he could wear his partial denture during breakfast and lunch?" I wondered.

In August, family members of the residents were invited to a newly formed Family Support Group that would meet monthly. The first meeting would be held on August 14, 2003. That meeting never materialized. The group disintegrated before it even got off the ground.

Trying to rein in Mark's smoking habit was an ongoing battle. In September, Mark signed an agreement that was intended to help him gain control of his smoking. The Unit Manager was to purchase one carton of cigarettes per month for Mark. They would then be distributed to him, one at a time, from the nurses' station (not to exceed SIX cigarettes per day. Suggested times were 9 a.m., noon, 2 p.m., 6 p.m., plus one time of Mark's choosing. The procedure was to be:

1) Mark would request a cigarette at the nurses' station.
2) Before he was given a cigarette, Mark would agree to use the bathroom. (Staff personnel would observe and document Mark's use of the bathroom.)
3) Mark would return to the nurses' station to get a cigarette.
4) Additionally, Mark would agree to refrain from asking members of the staff or residents for free cigarettes.
5) The document was signed by Mark and two witnesses.

I also created a chart with 5 columns–one for the day and date, one for the time of day, a column which listed cigarettes (numbered from one through six), a column for the bathroom, and a column for a staff member to acknowledge.

Day/Date	Time	Cigarette #	Bathroom Yes/No	Observed Sign/Initial
Th 9/11/03	9:00 am	1		
	Noon	2		
	2:00 pm	3		
	4:00 pm	4		
	6:00 pm	5		
	Other	6		
Fri 9/12/03	9:00 am	1		
	Noon	2		

The good news: By the end of October, the smoking schedule was working well. The rules had been modified; Mark had assumed responsibility for going to the bathroom before smoking (and remained continent), and the number of cigarettes was increased to eight. It was a win-win situation.

The bad news: The sliding door to the smoking area was difficult to open, and the ramp outside the door was unsafe. Several residents' wheelchairs had tipped and nearly toppled over the edge. The door and ramp needed to be repaired so they would meet safety codes.

Mark received this email from his best friend, Roz, on October 7, 2003:

TO A KEEPER.........

It was a way of life, and sometimes it made me crazy. All that re-fixing, reheating, renewing, I wanted just once to be wasteful. Waste meant affluence. Throwing things away meant you knew there'd always be more.

But then my Mother died, and on that clear, hot afternoon, in the warmth of the hospital room, I was struck with the pain of learning that sometimes there isn't anymore. No more hugs, no more special moments to celebrate together, no more phone calls just to chat, no more "just one minute." Sometimes, what we care about the most gets all used up and goes away...never to return before we can say goodbye, say "I love you."

So, while we have it...it's best we love it...and care for it... and fix it when it's broken...and heal it when it's sick.

This is true...for marriage...and old cars...and children with bad report cards...and dogs with bad hips...and aging parents... and grandparents...and friendships.

We keep them because they are worth it, because we are worth it. Some things we keep. Like a best friend that moved away. There are just some things that make us happy, no matter what, or a classmate we grew up with. Life is important, like people we know who are special...and so, we keep them close...in thought, in prayer, in deed.

I received this from someone who thought I was a 'keeper'! Then I sent it to people I think of in the same way. Now it's your turn to send this to all those people that are "keepers" in your life... like you!!

Thank you for being a special part of my life!
You're a Keeper!

"I long to accomplish a great and noble task, but it is my chief duty to accomplish small tasks as if they were great and noble"...Helen Keller

Mark sent this on to his dad Denny, his sister Lynn, his Uncle Gary, and his mom Colleen.

When I arrived at noon on October 15, 2003, Mark was sitting in his wheelchair, his clothing soaked with enema water, and he had had a bowel movement in his sweatpants. Mark's caretakers had given him an enema but did not provide him with a bedpan or make arrangements to get him to the bathroom afterward. It was disappointing how very little the CNAs knew—or what little training they had.

In December 2003, the residents' family members were invited to attend a monthly Resident/Family Advocate Group. The first meeting was to be on Thursday, December 11th, at 7:00 p.m. I looked forward to attending the meetings. Perhaps complaints would be addressed and resolved.

Mark's restorative therapy had been discontinued for nearly a month before I was informed. He had been receiving RT on Monday, Wednesday, and Friday. I had been giving Mark PT on Tuesday and Thursday when I visited him on my lunch break from work. Had I known his RT had been discontinued, I would have given him PT every day instead of just two days per week!

The year 2004 began with a new administrator. A few problems had been resolved or partially resolved. Maintenance received a repair order on January 26th to have the door and ramp to the smoking area repaired so residents could safely enter and exit. Mark's choking at mealtime was being monitored by the speech therapist. The toilet seat in the bathroom was fixed. However, when Mark entered the bathroom in his wheelchair, the door would not close, so he had no privacy and could not wash his hands. There were no suggestions for privacy, but Mark was provided hand cleanser as a substitute for washing his hands. Weeks after the physical therapy parallel bars were reported unstable, they were finally tightened.

The first Family Council Meeting (FCM) was held on February 12, 2004. Six family members, two residents, the administrator, and the social worker attended. We discussed our concerns and made suggestions for improvements. I kept records of each meeting, noting if the problems were resolved, partially resolved, or unresolved.

Six family members, one resident, and the activity director were at the March FCM. Two visitors gave presentations, one from Communications Systems and one from Samaritan Care Hospice. Of the previous meeting's concerns, four were partially resolved, and one was unresolved. Two new problems were added.

By Mark's April 20, 2004, Care Plan Meeting, his previous issues had been partially resolved. Staff seemed to be struggling to complete resident requests. I added the suggestion that Mark have his teeth and partial denture cleaned in the mornings before he went to breakfast.

Another new administrator came on board in May. Mark added a portable AM/FM CD Boombox to his inventory and also got a new harmonica, which helped to improve his breathing. He sincerely loved his music.

Attendance at the May 2004 Family Council Meeting (FCM) had dwindled to three family members, one resident, and the activity assistant. The list of concerns increased from 6 to 11. Of them, only one issue had been resolved. All prior problems were still partially resolved or unresolved. Several of them were re-submitted.

In June 2004, attendance at the FCM increased to 17 and included the new administrator, the ombudsman, and the council leader. The list of concerns had ballooned to 30. The major issues were unanswered call lights, oxygen supplies that were not being replaced, incontinent residents not being changed, flies in bathrooms, improper Foley catheter care, staff inexperience with lift chairs, broken lifts, no hot water or towels, whirlpool not working, and medicines not distributed on time. Even though an ombudsman was available, I learned early-on how ineffective they were. They were unable to address issues or solve problems and did not appear to be advocates of the residents. Instead, they identified more closely with the nursing home staff.

Issues discussed at Mark's Care Plan Meeting in July 2004 were gradually being addressed. Partial resolution seemed to be the norm. With my frequent visits to Mark, I could intercept significant problems and help with his care, so his stay at The Village would continue on at an acceptable level.

Numerous times over the years, in other nursing homes, I had attempted to have Mark's chart updated with accurate information. In August 2004, I made the request again at The Village. His chart depicted him as paraplegic (paralyzed from the waist down). Mark was not paralyzed in any way. His chart also denoted that he had high blood pressure even though Mark's blood pressure was well within the normal range. I was never successful in having his chart corrected.

On December 2, 2004, I sent an email to the new administrator to let him know about the bathroom problems:

1) Bathroom access posed a safety hazard due to lack of room.

2) Unsanitary conditions existed, since most often the urine and feces ended up on the floor, instead of in the toilet.

3) Mark was unable to reach the sink to wash his hands.

4) There was a lack of privacy since both the bathroom door and the room door could not be closed. When I visited Mark between noon and 1:00 p.m., three staff members were using his room to eat, retrieve items from Mark's roommate's refrigerator, and store their coats.

Five days later, Mark was moved into a different room (his fourth since he was admitted in July of 2002). However, some of the old problems remained with him, and others were exchanged for new ones. I asked his new caretakers to schedule Mark to use the bathroom first thing in the morning and the last thing before he went to bed at night to help him remain continent. Later, when I visited Mark at lunchtime, he was in bed, with the side rails up, so he couldn't get out of bed. His new caretakers didn't understand that Mark could transfer from his bed to his wheelchair without assistance. Spilled food remained on the floor overnight. Two work orders remained unfulfilled: one was for the closet pole to be lowered so Mark could reach his clothes, and the other was to replace the towel bar in the bathroom. (The bar and fixtures were on the shelf under the sink in the bathroom.)

After a third request, the work orders were completed on January 3, 2005. There were three family members, two residents, and the council president at the January 13, 2005, FCM. Five of the concerns were resolved, several were partially resolved, and others remained unresolved.

Mark's January 18, 2005, Care Plan Meeting went smoothly. Most of his needs were being addressed, although caretakers still needed to be reminded of Mark's ability to help himself. The activity director set up times for Mark and his chess-playing partner to play.

At the end of the month, I delivered a new magnetic chess set to Mark. That made it much easier for him to play since his lack of hand coordination would sometimes push the chessmen off the board.

Problems with loss of clothing in the laundry department had been ongoing since Mark arrived at The Village. Family Council Volunteers had begun typing labels for the residents' clothing when the facilities director left the department. Plans for the volunteers to iron on the labels went astray when she left, and the laundry was outsourced.

The status of the Family Council's concerns remained unchanged in the February meeting. Two new situations were added. Even though the nursing director and the council president attended the meeting, the issues apparently were not reaching those with the authority to implement solutions. It's as though we were spinning our wheels, and the discussions were for naught.

Saturday, February 19, 2005, Mark was admitted to Baylor Richardson Medical Center with a recurring fever. I visited Mark twice on Monday – before I went to work and at 5:45 p.m. That morning I asked that Mark be given a denture cup for his partial denture and asked that he have his teeth brushed. During my second visit, I found that fluids had leaked from his IV, all over his sheets, gown, and pillow where his arm was resting. He had also wet his diaper and was soaked with urine. The nurse said she would clean Mark after she took care of another patient. A second nurse came by and helped with Mark. When the first nurse returned, I asked her about Mark's denture cup. She had forgotten. When I asked if anyone had helped Mark on the bedside commode, they hadn't. When Mark's dinner tray came, the menu clearly stated, "ground meat;" however, a big pork steak was on the plate. We made the decision that Mark should be served a puree diet. At least, he couldn't choke on that! I erroneously believed that the hospital's care would be better than the care in the nursing home. Seeing this neglect in the medical field was utterly disappointing and totally unacceptable.

Mark was moved back to The Village on February 23, 2005. Things were unchanged. At the March 10, 2005, Family Council meeting, all of the partially resolved issues from the list of concerns were removed; they would never be totally resolved. Seven unresolved issues remained. March 10, 2005, was my last record of the Family Council Meetings. Only two residents, two family members, and the activity director had attended. Due to lack of action, the group had gradually disintegrated.

I sent memos to the unit manager on three separate occasions: March 21st, 24th, and 31st. When I visited Mark on March 21st, he had an empty breathing treatment apparatus in his mouth, was soaked with urine, his teeth were not brushed, his partial denture was still in the cup in the bathroom, and he had not shaved. On March 24, 2005, Mark's bed was not locked in place, dirty laundry was left on the floor of his closet, and when OT picked up Mark for therapy, he was soaked with urine. On March 31, 2005, I explained that when I visited Mark on March 30th, a tooth was missing from his partial denture, and the denture was lying on his bedside table, instead of in its cup. Caretakers and I searched extensively for the missing tooth but were unable to find it. I asked that a dental appointment be made so Mark could have his denture repaired or replaced.

On March 31, 2005, the administrator was replaced by an interim administrator. By the end of April, a former administrator returned to The Village. He had been at The Village when Mark moved there in July of 2002. It was interesting how the administrators seemed to be playing a game of "Musical Chairs."

A new psychologist began meeting with Mark in April 2005. Dr. X wanted to change the focus of his therapy. She recognized Mark's potential for higher-level activities and responsibilities by playing chess with him. She covered topics that others had not touched upon and spoke honestly with Mark regarding his future. Because Mark's speech was sometimes difficult to understand, his psychologist was patient and encouraged him to use his voice. Dr. X reminded him to greet others and thank them for the care they provided for him and saw that Mark followed through. I was impressed with how she interacted with Mark. She treated him with respect and saw him as an individual–not just another nursing home resident. She learned the type of music he liked to listen to and brought him travel magazines to spark his interest. Mark had been in hospitals, rehab facilities, and nursing homes since his head injury in 1994. It was inspiring to encounter such an optimistic person as she, with her fresh ideas and positive outlook for her patients. I sent a letter to her clinical director, commending her for her outstanding work.

Mark's roommate could not comprehend boundaries. When Mark received a new denture cup, his roommate continued to put his dentures in it. His urinal was usually sitting on his bedside chest, directly next to Mark's computer table. I asked that it be emptied more often or, at least, moved into the bathroom. He would often place his items on Mark's bedside table instead of his own. The dresser upon which his television sat was shoved against Mark's dresser so forcefully that it displaced Mark's guitar that was hanging on the wall. His roommate tried to make a plastic cup holder fit on the arm of his wheelchair. To enlarge it, he held the flame from his cigarette lighter to it to soften the plastic – a dangerous fire and safety hazard – and I was considering how I would put out the fire if the plastic began to burn. I sent a memo to the unit manager and asked her to address the issues.

On April 20, 2005, Mark's computer was moved out of his room while the floors were stripped and waxed. When it was reconnected the next day by the maintenance man, it didn't work. The administrator looked at the computer and assured me that it would be fixed. A week later, I sent the administrator a memo asking him to arrange to have it fixed as soon as possible. On May 6, 2005, I tried unsuccessfully to repair the operating system from the software CD. Finally, on May 19, 2005, I hired a PC repairman who had to replace the hard drive and operating system, which had been corrupted. Mark had been without his computer for a month. The Village agreed to pay for the repairs, but I did not receive a check from them until August.

Although I had sent documentation of ongoing issues to both the administrator and unit manager in May, many of the problems were worse. Because little was being done to correct them, I addressed and resolved them myself. New problems kept cropping up with his roommate: he continued to use Mark's chest of drawers and bed for his belongings, did not clean up after himself when he used the bathroom, and would not throw away old food. I visited Mark nearly every day on my lunch break from work, and each time I needed to clean his room when I would have preferred to spend more quality time with him.

At 6:00 a.m. on June 2, 2005, I received a call from Mark's nurse, letting me know that Mark had fallen in the bathroom. Even though she assured me that he was all right, I left for The Village right away to check on him. Up until then, Mark had been transferring from his wheelchair to the toilet without incident. When I arrived, I discovered that the toilet seat extension was totally askew and not securely attached to the toilet. The prior week, the unit manager and I had discussed replacing the toilet seat extension because it was both dirty and loose. Two previous memos addressing these issues that had been sent to the administrator, dated May 17th and May 27th, went unheeded.

At Mark's care plan meeting on June 6, 2005, all previously unresolved issues were discussed and were on their way to being resolved. It had been nearly three months since Mark's partial denture had been broken; the estimated date of resolution for this was September 5th.

More memos were sent or faxed to the administrator in early June. There continued to be multiple issues that created safety and health hazards. Shoes and socks were placed next to Mark's toothbrush; food, drink, and Mark's CD player were left on the bathroom counter; and there were feces all over the toilet seat. And then, on June 12th, Mark's nurse called me to tell me that his denture was broken and missing. That evening, I went to The Village and found a piece of it lying on the bathroom counter. The remaining broken denture was discovered in Mark's mouth; I retrieved it and took it home.

Could it possibly get any worse? Apparently, it could. Two days later, during my noon visit, I found liquid and discarded towels covered in feces on the floor. Mark's roommate's full urinal was hanging on his bed rail, and a carton of milk had been sitting on his bedside table since morning. I had to shoo the flies away from Mark's dinner tray while he ate his dinner.

The following Wednesday, Mark's roommate's urinal was sitting directly on Mark's tray table, where he ate his meals. The table was wet beneath the urinal. Two of his roommate's cups with liquid in them were sitting on Mark's chest and his washcloth, covered with feces, was on the bathroom floor. I again faxed my concerns to the administrator, reminding him that we had been discussing this situation for several weeks. Even after holding an additional Care Plan Meeting on June 6th, it appeared there had been no communication to the staff to correct these hazardous and totally unacceptable conditions. I let him know that I was weary of observing those unsanitary conditions on a daily basis and requested that his roommate be moved out of Mark's room. I asked him what he thought the State would say about this situation. Not an hour after I sent the fax, the administrator called to tell me that Mark would be relocated to the 1400 Hall.

On June 30, 2005, I received a call from the assistant administrator telling me that *an ember from Mark's cigarette fell on his leg*, burned a hole in his clothing, and left *a red mark on his leg*. She told me that Mark would be re-assessed for safe smoking. Since smoking was supposed to be supervised, I wondered what happened. That incident would be the beginning of subsequent occurrences of **CIGARETTE BURNS**. Mark's smoking apron was in shreds and needed to be replaced. His caretakers used the apron as a bib when he ate his meals, because they did not know its purpose.

Before Mark could be moved to a different room, he hit his roommate. After the confrontation, the roommate was moved at his request, and Mark's psychiatrist increased his Zyprexa to prevent any further outbursts.

Before leaving for vacation on August 13, 2005, I left a battery charger and four new rechargeable batteries with the unit managers so Mark could be assisted with changing batteries in his CD player. I left a list of detailed instructions in the unit manager's office, the nurse's station, and the front desk. When I returned from vacation on Monday, August 22, 2005, Mark's CD batteries had not been changed since I left—over a week before. In his battery charger, which was still plugged into the wall in the unit manager's office, were two non-rechargeable batteries. The unit manager was no longer working at The Village, and since the current one could not locate the missing rechargeable batteries, she replaced them with non-rechargeable ones. I intervened, and the administrator replaced the rechargeable batteries.

Mark had been released from restorative therapy several weeks before I learned about the change. The CNAs were to pick up his therapy but didn't. After notifying the administrator, I was told it would begin

Monday, August 29, 2005.

It seemed that the only way to get anything done was to contact the administrator. Both zippered cases containing Mark's scissors and nail clippers were missing from his drawer, and the armrest from his wheelchair needed to be replaced; after I notified the administrator (again), both were replaced. Mark had lab tests for blood in his anal area in July and was seen by a specialist in August, who asked that Mark be monitored; I had to report the bleeding again at the end of September at his Care Plan Meeting, though, because the CNAs did not follow through. I later made another appointment for him to see a specialist.

On October 6th, Mark had surgery to repair an anal fistula at Medical City Plano. The colon prep was so poorly done at The Village that Mark was admitted to the hospital the day before his surgery, so the prep could be redone there. I kept a close watch on him when he returned to The Village to ensure the post-op instructions were carried out properly. The surgery was successful, and Mark was healing nicely. Mark's lost denture, which I had first discussed with staff, was to be replaced around September 5th. Mark's new social worker could find no documentation regarding the denture, though. The documents were resubmitted on September 6, 2005, and the revised estimated date of confirmation or denial would be October 7, 2005.

In January 2006, Mark's quality of care continued to decline. In yet another memo to the administrator on January 4th, I stressed how Mark's **CIGARETTE BURN ON HIS RIGHT THIGH** was not being cared for properly. He had been incontinent, and **THE BANDAGE WAS SOAKED WITH URINE AND STUCK TO THE BURN.** The wound care nurse was on vacation, and no one had bothered to change the dressing while he was away.

A leg brace had been delivered to Mark's room, however, PT had not evaluated him for it. It had been over a month since Restorative Therapy informed the PT department of Mark's need to be evaluated. I asked the administrator to please check into PT's schedule and see that

Mark be evaluated as soon as possible.

Here is an email that I sent to the social worker on March 3rd:

"Subject: Mark Ostrander 1612B. I just had another unpleasant visit to The Village today. I arrived at 1:25 p.m. Mark was ready to have a cigarette, so I asked him to go to the bathroom before he went out to smoke. He was soaked with urine–his underclothing, sweatpants, and both shirts he was wearing.

"It was 1:30 p.m. when I asked him to pull the emergency light in his bathroom. I waited for five minutes, and when no one came, I went to the nurses' station to see if someone was coming. I could hear the emergency alarm at the station, however, when I asked the person sitting at the desk, she said she could not identify which light was on, because the light board was broken, and it was not showing up on the board. She then alerted people to fix the board.

"I located Mark's caretaker, who accompanied me to Mark's room. By that time, ten minutes had elapsed from the time the emergency light was activated.

"This concerns me very much. Had I not gone to the nurses' station, I doubt that anyone would have answered Mark's call. It is totally unacceptable and very serious that an emergency light is not answered for ten minutes.

"Will you please see that the unit manager gets a copy of this email? She is the person who has implemented the bowel and bladder program for Mark, and it is apparently not being followed by her afternoon staff. Since I began visiting Mark later in the day, I have found him both wet and soiled more often than dry and clean. Wednesday evening when I visited Mark at 6:30 p.m., he was wet. His caretaker told me, 'He is going to have a shower this evening, anyway.' Apparently, she didn't understand that had she followed the program, Mark would not be wet. I keep getting excuses from the staff that Mark refuses to go to the bathroom. I told

them the next time he refuses, to please call me, and I will come and personally see that he does. So far, I have received no calls. Thanks for your help…Colleen Nuncio"

On the 15th, I sent the social worker another email:

"This is a request to either 1) train the night care person who is caring for Mark Ostrander, Room 1612B, or 2) assign a different night caretaker for him. When Mark's daytime caretaker arrives at work in the morning, she finds Mark's clothing and bed wet with urine. Mark is capable of using the toilet, and it has been requested that he use the toilet before he goes to bed, or during the night. Evidence shows that those instructions are not being followed. Tuesday morning, March 14, 2006, in addition to his being wet, she also found Mark's partial denture on the bathroom counter (not in the denture cup on his bedside chest, where it is supposed to be.) Occasionally, she finds Mark's denture still in his mouth in the morning, which indicates he has not received evening dental care. Dental care instructions are posted on the wall in Mark's room.

"In December 2005, Mark received a new partial denture that replaced his original one which was found broken on the floor of his room. It took nearly a year before he received his replacement.

"I asked the previous unit manager to learn which night employee was caring for Mark, so she could resolve these problems, but she did not take action. Will you please see that the new unit manager gets a copy of this email, so he can act upon this request? Thank you for your help…Colleen Nuncio"

All my pleas for improvement went unheeded, so mid-March 2006, I sent an email to the unit manager asking her to assign a different night caretaker to Mark. Requests that Mark use the bathroom before he went to bed had been disregarded; his bedding and clothing were found wet in the morning, and, occasionally Mark's denture was still in his mouth in the morning, indicating that dental care was not being given at bedtime even though dental care instructions were posted on the wall in Mark's room. Additionally, Mark was allowed to eat in his leather jacket and his smoking apron—they were filthy! A pureed diet was not being followed, and many times there was solid food on his tray.

By the time April arrived, I had discussed several unacceptable issues with the ombudsman. I noted the following in a fax to the administrator on Wednesday, April 19, 2006.

1. *The extended toilet seat in the bathroom was loose and unsafe.*
2. *Mark's clothing was soaked with urine*
3. *Mark's partial denture was not in his mouth.*

The ombudsman said he would bring these issues to your attention on Monday. Yesterday, April 18, 2006, I visited Mark at 6:00 p.m. The toilet seat in his bathroom was literally falling off. I called the unit manager to observe the seat. I also told him that I was not leaving until the seat was made safe. I easily lifted the seat off the toilet, as it was not attached. Then the unit manager and I searched and found a shower chair that we placed over the toilet.

A bowel and bladder program was to be in place to keep Mark continent. I had Mark at my home on Saturday and at my sister's home on Sunday. Both days, Mark remained continent. I only took him to the bathroom once.

You and I have discussed Mark's dental procedure many times in the past. To date, Mark's caretakers seem oblivious to this part of Mark's care.

Once again, I am weary of observing these unacceptable conditions on a daily basis when I visit my son. Do you have any solutions?

Thank you.

Colleen Nuncio, Mark Ostrander's Mother

I faxed a copy of this to Senior Source at the State of Texas Department of Aging and Disability Services.

Thank goodness for the weekends! Mark's cousin Laurie had moved to Texas from Minnesota in April 2006, and she became an important part of Mark's life and one of his biggest supporters. She lived with my sister, Joan, in the country in Emory, Texas. Frequently, Joan invited members of our family to visit on the weekend for a midday potluck. As much as Mark looked forward to the family gatherings, I remember one particular time we were driving to Joan's, and out of the blue, Mark said, "Kill me." Part of his life was missing, and how empty he must have felt!

Every year we celebrated Mark's birthday, which was April 29th. This evolved into a monthly group poolside birthday party at our house during the summer and fall when we would honor all the local relatives whose birthdays were that particular month. Although the number of guests dwindled over the years as our relatives moved away, we continued to bring Mark to our house on the weekends. When it was warm, we helped him walk in the pool to strengthen his muscles and improve his balance.

Over the course of 5 days, between May 18th and May 22nd, I sent faxes to the administrator, the ombudsman, and Senior Source outlining, once again, issues with Mark's menu, a broken pull chain in the bathroom, the filthy toilet seat, and the poor personal care he was receiving. I hoped they would begin to finally see that the staff was neglectful and not providing proper standards of care, and patients were suffering for it.

I sent another fax on May 23rd and, in addition to the earlier issues, I alerted the recipients to a **LARGE BLISTER ON THE SECOND FINGER OF MARK'S RIGHT HAND**, where he held his cigarettes. I asked the unit manager to observe the burn and dried feces that were stuck to his bottom. She mentioned that Mark may need to be supervised when he smoked, and had Mark's caretaker clean him.

Two days later, I faxed to the administrator, ombudsman, and Senior Source that the **BLISTER ON MARK'S FINGER HAD BROKEN OPEN**. The wound and Mark's hands were filthy. I had Mark wash his hands and asked the nurse for a Band-Aid to put on the open blister. He applied an ointment to the wound and covered it with a Band-Aid. Mark's room and body were clean during this visit. I thanked the administrator for his involvement in Mark's care.

Alas! It didn't last. The next day the unsanitary bathroom and smoking apron issues were once again apparent.

An email that I sent to the social worker (administrator copied) on May 30th, notifying them that the armrest was missing from Mark's wheelchair, was responded to the next day, noting that the armrest had arrived and was being installed. Hooray! Action was taken when the request was directed to the appropriate people!

On June 1, 2006, I emailed the administrator to let him know that Mark's restorative therapist told me that Mark would not receive therapy after June 1st. He indicated that Mark would need to be re-evaluated to continue. He said that Mark had shown progress, which, I thought, was a prerequisite for Mark to continue therapy. I requested he arrange to have Mark re-evaluated for RT.

When I arrived to pick up Mark on Sunday, June 4th, he was coming down the hall in his wheelchair and was soaked with urine. Also, the water in the toilet tank in Mark's bathroom was running, and the toilet could not be flushed. I jiggled the handle several times, and it would not stop running. I informed two staff members of the problem. When no one came to clean Mark after 20 minutes, I took care of it, using washcloths and a pillowcase since there were no towels on the linen cart.

Before we left, I asked Mark's caretaker to make a copy of Mark's smoking schedule. She knew nothing about his schedule and could not locate the copy that had been at the nurses' station.

When we returned that evening, the water in the toilet tank was still running. I told the supervisor and let him know I had informed the staff earlier. I was so upset when I found that the toilet could not be fixed. I sent an email to the administrator from Mark's computer before leaving.

The next day, Monday, June 5th, I sent an email from my computer to the administrator, ombudsman, and Senior Source, listing what I had found when I visited at 11:45 a.m.:

1. The water in the toilet tank was still running (since the day before), the toilet could not be flushed, and the bowl was filling up with toilet paper.
2. There were feces all over the toilet seat, and Mark had feces on his clothing.
3. There was food on the floor (spinach) that had been there since yesterday's lunch. The DON and East Side nurse observed the situation. I informed them that I had asked three staff members to correct the situation yesterday and asked if the staff was aware there are maintenance workers onsite on Sunday. I was told they would submit a work request; however, when the DON and I spoke with two people from Maintenance, both said they had not been informed of the situation. I also sent this email to Texas Congressman Sam Johnson in the House of Representatives, Washington D.C. I asked him to direct me to a process or a "next step" that would convince the nursing home it must improve conditions and provide satisfactory care. I found no record of response to this email.

On June 6th I sent this email:

Hello, Administrator,

I'm sure you are getting tired of receiving these unpleasant emails from me. I am getting tire of sending them to you, but I feel that I need to report to you the inadequate care my son is receiving.

Today, I visited Mark at 11:30 a.m. When Mark used the bathroom, I observed feces in and on his clothing and covering his bottom and legs. The unit manager observed the situation and arranged for Mark's caregiver to clean Mark.

Are the caregivers not taking your requests seriously? Since they should be aware of Mark's schedule by now, why can't they follow a simple instruction to have Mark adhere to a two-hour bathroom schedule? It would seem a lot easier to clean Mark after he has used the toilet, than to have to clean him after he has a bowel movement and pulls up his pants without wiping. If not, could they at least check him periodically to see if he needs attention?

In my June 7th email to the administrator that I sent at 12:03 p.m., I informed him that Mark's toilet could not be flushed because the chain had fallen into the tank and was no longer connected to the handle. I received an email from the administrator less than 10 minutes later, letting me know that it had been repaired. What a nice and timely response!

In a June 12th email, I asked the administrator the status of my request for Mark's restorative therapy evaluation. The next day, he emailed this explanation:

"Mark's progress towards the last restorative nursing goals reached the limits of his potential. He has not declined to any point that he would benefit from additional restorative therapy at this time. Mark has been on the restorative programs for over a year. Most programs conclude at the three-month time frame. We will keep our eyes on him for future potential."

By July, the administrator was no longer at The Village. The assistant administrator had taken his place. Conditions were becoming intolerable, so my first email to her, sent Monday, July 10th, was lengthy and replete with unsatisfactory practices.

Today was one of the worst visits I have experienced in the four years that Mark has been a resident. I arrived around 12:40 p.m. Plans were to help Mark with weight-bearing exercise, have him use the bathroom, and get him to his smoking area by 1:00 p.m.

Lunch arrived when I was there, so he quickly finished lunch and, when he went into the bathroom, I observed dried feces in his groin area. (His bottom was clean.) I asked the unit manager if she could get someone to clean Mark. She referred me to the new nurse, who observed the feces (and blood) in Mark's diaper and said she would get Mark's caregiver to clean him. Ten minutes later, Mark was still sitting on the toilet, waiting for his caregiver. I told the nurse, and she personally went to the dining area to get the caregiver. Twenty minutes later, when no one came, I reminded the nurse; she told me that the caregiver was busy and unable to come, so she would find someone else. I once again reminded the unit manager that Mark was still waiting.

Thirty-five minutes later, Mark's caretaker came to his room and told me she had to go to the laundry to get towels. Then she told me the laundry would not allow her to get any towels. I retrieved a sheet and a pillowcase from the laundry cart and was going to clean Mark when, miraculously, she found some towels.

The caretaker was totally unhappy with the situation, and when I asked her if she had observed the blood in Mark's diaper, she said that she had. I told her that it was from a surgical incision and that when she cleaned Mark's bottom, she needed to be gentle so it would not re-open the wound. When I asked her to look at the wound, she refused, and told me that was the nurse's job, not hers. I asked the nurse to document the caretaker's uncooperative response. (The nurse thought the blood was coming from Mark's penis; however, she did not even examine him. I have no idea how she documented it.)

It was after 1:30 p.m. when Mark was ready for his cigarette that he had missed at 1:00 p.m. I asked the unit manager if she could make an exception, and I would monitor Mark while he smoked. She stated that she had to go by the rules and could not do that. That was when I met you and asked if you could make the exception, and you agreed to call the unit manager.

I went to Mark's room, retrieved his smoking apron, and stopped to pick up a cigarette at the nurse's station on my way to the smoking area. The unit manager told me that someone had already taken Mark to the smoking area and would supervise him. I asked, "Without his smoking apron?" She replied that she thought he was wearing his smoking apron. I told her she couldn't just "think" he was wearing it–she needed to confirm that he had it on.

I'm willing to help in any way that I can to make your staff's job easier. Today, members of the East Wing staff were rude and unprofessional.

On Saturday, I experienced the same non-cooperation when I arrived at The Village at 4:00 p.m. The nurse tried to locate Mark's caregiver and have him clean Mark, whose diaper was full of feces. When he couldn't locate the caregiver, he commented that the staff members hide when they are needed and try to get out of the work.

It seems that morale is very low, and the staff takes no interest in doing a decent job. I know how difficult it must be for you to organize a situation that seems so out of control, but something needs to be done to improve these circumstances. Thank you for any help you can provide....Colleen Nuncio

The very next day, July 11th, at 2:47 p.m., I sent another email to the nurse:

Today no one was in the smoking area to provide the residents with cigarettes at 1:00 p.m. At 1:30 p.m., I asked who was scheduled to supervise the smoking today; the unit manager told me it was the Maintenance Department. She called Maintenance, and they informed her that they had other things to do at that time. They also told her that they had not informed anyone, nor had they arranged for someone else to assume the responsibility.

When I left The Village at 1:45 p.m., she was still trying to delegate the task.

If the staff implements new procedures and sets new rules for the residents, they need to uphold their side of the bargain and follow through with their promises…Colleen Nuncio

At 4:23 p.m., I received an email from the caregiver. She apologized for the delay and informed me that the residents were able to smoke. She stated, "We will try to improve quickly."

On Tuesday, July 25, 2006, at 10:39 a.m., I faxed the following to the administrator.

At 8:00 a.m. on Sunday, July 23, 2006, I called The Village to let the nurse know that I would be there to pick up Mark at 9:00 a.m.

At 9:05 a.m., when I arrived at The Village, Mark's caretaker could not be located. I found Mark in his room, in bed, still in his gown, soaked with urine. I promptly got him up and took him to the shower room. The shower room floor had pools of water on the floor, and the shower chair had to be cleaned. After soaking up the water and cleaning the shower chair, I began to shower Mark. Soon Mark's caretaker came into the shower room, and together we showered Mark, brushed his teeth, shaved him, combed his hair, and got him ready to leave.

I DISCOVERED A DIME-SIZED BLISTER ON THE INSTEP OF MARK'S LEFT FOOT. I COULD SEE WHERE

HIS SHOE HAD BEEN BURNED FROM A DROPPED CIGARETTE ASH. I asked that the burn be documented. The wound was not dressed, although Mark's caretaker said he had noticed the burn earlier in the week. It should have been reported.

When I returned Mark to The Village after 8 o'clock that evening, I asked Mark's caregiver who would be supervising the 9 o'clock smoking. He shouted disrespectfully the length of the hall to ask another caregiver. This was not the first time Mark's caregiver acted inappropriately. In the past, he lied to me and contradicted information that his fellow staff members had provided me, which I knew to be accurate. You may want to act upon this information that I have shared with you…Colleen Nuncio

Friday, July 28, 2006, I emailed to the administrator:

Yesterday, Thursday, July 27, 2006, when I visited Mark at 5:30 p.m., he was sitting in the smoking area. I asked him if he had eaten, and he said he had not. We went to his room; his lunch tray was still sitting on his tray table. I put his lunch tray on the cart in the hall and took his dinner tray from the cart into his room.

Before he ate, he was going to use the bathroom. I noticed there were feces on the toilet seat. There were also feces in his pants. Instead of sitting on the toilet, I had Mark begin eating his dinner while I contacted his nurse to have someone clean Mark and the bathroom.

Mark's caretaker was unavailable so Nurse asked Caretaker to help with Mark. I pointed out that Mark was to use the bathroom every two hours (sign on the wall of Mark's room). Caretaker stated that she couldn't interrupt a resident while he was eating, to which I agreed. I also informed her of the lunch tray still in Mark's room at 5:30 pm. She began to raise her voice, telling me why his tray was still there; I asked her please not to use that tone of voice. Nurse observed this exchange.

I asked Nurse who would be supervising the 6 p.m. smoking. According to the schedule, someone from the 1300 hall and the 2500 hall were scheduled. Nurse told me that the 1300 hall caretaker was busy and could not supervise, so she got a volunteer to take Mark for his 6 p.m. cigarette. The nurse and volunteer were unable to locate Mark's cigarettes; a second nurse joined in the search. (This same thing happened last week. After 15 minutes of searching, his cigarettes were found by the activities director and placed in the medication room, where she asked that they stay.) Nurse #2 looked in the medication room and stated she could not find them and that Mark had probably smoked them all. She also told me that the smoking schedule signs were wrong and that the 6:00 p.m. smoking had been moved to 6:45 p.m.

Mark and I returned to the outside smoking area, where several residents were waiting for the 6 p.m. monitor to arrive. At 6:20 p.m., I returned to the nurse's station and told them that the residents were waiting for the person who supervises the smoking. When I returned to the smoking area, two activity directors (ADs) were walking into the facility. I told them about Mark's missing cigarettes and the missing smoking supervisor. At that time, AD #1 announced over the PA system that the smoking supervisor needed to go to the smoking area immediately. The ADs personally went to the med room and located Mark's carton of cigarettes. When I mentioned the new smoking time, both ADs said that neither they nor the residents had been informed of this.

I try not to report every little incident to you. (Earlier this week, when I visited at lunchtime, Mark's breakfast tray was still sitting in his room. I removed it before I placed his lunch tray on the tray table and did not report it.) I know that the caretakers become very busy at times, but every day?

Is there anything you can do to have these situations corrected? ...Colleen Nuncio

Desperate to find improvements to the shoddy care of the NH residents, I sent my next email to the Director of Consumer Rights and Services (DCRS), Texas Department of Aging and Disability Services (DADS) on Wednesday, August 2, 2006 at 3:52 p.m.

Dear DCRS,

*Today, when I visited my son, Mark Ostrander, at The Village at Richardson Nursing Home in Richardson TX, I was fortunate to meet your Department of Aging and Disabilities Representative (Rep). I showed her the **CIGARETTE BURNS THAT ARE ON MARK'S FOOT AND LEG.** After discussing the many unacceptable practices that have been occurring at The Village, Rep advised me to contact you and inform you of the inadequate care my son has been receiving.*

I have been emailing my observations and requests to The Village Administrator(s), hoping that improvements would be made. Unfortunately, Mark's care is deteriorating, and each day that I visit, I become more frustrated. I will forward to you the emails that I sent to the administrator(s) in July through August 1, 2006. If you are unable to act upon that information, I will provide you with previous observations and requests that I have communicated to the administrator(s).

The subject of the emails I will send to you will be: Mark Ostrander 1612B. When you have read them, can you please take action to see that these conditions improve?

I look forward to your response.

Regards,

Colleen Nuncio

Mark Ostrander's Mother

I forwarded all the emails to the DCRS that I had sent to the administrator from June 26, 2006 through August 3, 2006.

Monday, August 7th, at 10:36 a.m., I sent the following email to the DCRS.

> *On Saturday (August 5th), the DADS representatives from Arlington, TX, visited The Village Nursing Home to observe their smoking practices. Later that day, the Director of Nursing called to inform me that the State had visited, and due to the very serious allegations regarding smoking, The Village was implementing some changes to their smoking policy. She said that Mark would have his cigarette held by a staff member while he smoked.*
>
> *On Sunday evening, the unit manager called me and read to me the conditions of the new policy. Later, she called to tell me that Mark had violated the conditions of the policy, and she had given him a warning that upon his second violation, he would be discharged from the facility.*
>
> *Mark's violation: He was in the smoking area, and a resident (who should not have had cigarettes) gave Mark a cigarette, which he smoked. I have repeatedly asked the residents not to give Mark cigarettes and informed them that he is allowed only one cigarette during smoking times. Mark has no cigarettes in his possession.*
>
> *It looks like Mark is going to need an advocate or legal counsel to help him in his terrible situation. What do you recommend that he do?*
>
> *Thank you for all your help…Colleen Nuncio*

That same day, the DADS representative submitted another complaint to the regional office for the surveyors to investigate. She mentioned that it could be *Retaliation.*

The Village personnel were not happy with me for informing the State of the intolerable conditions! It was my understanding that, after the State's inspection, The Village was fined on a daily basis until they became compliant with all the State's rules and regulations. Needless to say, The Village would try their best to get rid of Mark.

Monday, August 7th, Mark received a letter via hand delivery from The Village.

Re: Violation of Smoking Policy

Dear Mr. Ostrander:

As you are aware, our nursing facility recently instituted a new smoking policy whereby all residents must be supervised while they smoke. I have been advised that, despite verbal direction and warning, you violated this policy on Sunday, August 6, 2006, by borrowing a cigarette from another resident and smoking without supervision.

This correspondence shall serve as written warning that, in the event you violate this policy in the future, we will be left with no other choice but to prepare a safe discharge plan for your transfer from this facility. While we truly hope this is not necessary, our facility has an obligation to provide each resident with a safe living environment. Violations of our smoking policy pose a risk and danger to others and, as such, cannot be permitted.

We hope you will reconsider your refusal to abide by this policy and appreciate your anticipated cooperation in protecting our residents.

Please feel free to contact me if you wish to discuss this matter further.

Sincerely,

____

Facility Administrator

It wasn't long before Mark had his second smoking violation and received notice that he would be discharged. On September 15, 2006, Mark moved to Elm Fork Nursing and Rehab in Carrollton, TX.

CHAPTER 13

Too Dangerous to Disregard
September 15, 2006–July 15, 2008

ON MY LUNCH break each day, I would make the nearly one-hour drive to Elm Fork Nursing and Rehab in Carrollton, Texas, and back. I was fortunate to have a very caring and compassionate boss who understood my dilemma and provided me the time to be with Mark.

We became quite proficient in moving Mark from nursing home to nursing home. With each move, I would familiarize the caretakers with Mark's capabilities and routines.

On Monday, September 18, 2006, three days after Mark moved to Elm Fork, at 1:30 in the afternoon, I found Mark in bed with the rails up, even though he could transfer from his bed to his wheelchair on his own. His teeth had not been brushed, even though his electric toothbrush was in full view, and his partial denture was still in a cup. He was unshaven, even though his electric shaver was in plain sight. He was wearing diapers with tape closures–not the pull-ups that enabled him to conveniently use the bathroom. A bag of dirty laundry was on a chair in his room. I gave the assistant administrator (AA) my list of observations and apprised him of Mark's abilities and his needs.

I accompanied Mark to the smoking area where the monitor was talking on her cell phone. She ignored me when I tried to point out to her that Mark had arrived. Although it was her responsibility, I proceeded to put a smoking apron on Mark, lit his cigarette for him, and supervised him while he smoked. I made sure he smoked slowly and that he intermittently put his ashes in the ashtray. Before I left Elm Fork later that day, I reported the unprofessional actions of the smoking monitor to the AA.

When I arrived at work on Tuesday morning, I had messages from Elm Fork asking me to call the nursing home. This happened again the following Friday. I wondered why they would call me after my working hours at my work number when they had my personal phone number.

During the month of September, I spent a lot of time teaching the staff how to care for Mark. Over and over, the same mistakes were made. When I needed to take Mark out, I would call well in advance and ask the staff to shower and shave him, as well as brush his teeth by a specific time; however, he would never be ready. When I arrived to pick him up on Sunday, September 24th, he was in the shower, although I had called well in advance. He was bleeding and draining from his surgical incision; the room was in total disarray, and the bathroom grab bar was broken. I reported the issues to the nurse. By the time we returned late that afternoon, the broken grab bar had been replaced.

On Thursday, September 28, 2006, the top part of Mark's electric toothbrush was missing. I reported it to the AA, along with the fact that Mark had no pull-up diapers. The AA promised that he would have pull-up diapers placed in Mark's room and would see that they would be used for Mark.

Saturday, September 30th, I took Mark a new brush for his electric toothbrush. He was lying in bed, soaked with urine. He was wearing taped diapers, even though there were pull-ups in his closet. I had to tell the CNA about the pull-ups; it seemed that communication between staff members needed some improvement. The CNA cleaned Mark while I stripped the sheets from his bed. Mark's hairbrush and electric shaver were missing. I reported the missing items to the activity director and the DON, then completed a grievance report, which I gave to the DON.

Mark's electric shaver had not been found by Monday, October 2nd, so I provided the staff with a picture of it and a receipt for its cost. I asked the CNA to please shave Mark with a disposable razor until the electric shaver was located. Mark was wearing taped diapers that were around his knees. Although the AA provided pull-ups for Mark, the business office personnel informed me that pull-ups were not provided; the family needed to purchase them. So I suggested that Mark be started on a bowel and bladder program, since he had previously been continent since his brain injury.

The AA requested that I email him regarding Mark's lost electric shaver. I repeated the request I had given to the CNA to please shave Mark with a disposable razor until his electric shaver was found or replaced. Mark hadn't been shaved since September 30th, when I noticed that his shaver was missing. It appeared that in order to get anything accomplished, I would need to communicate directly with the AA or the administrator.

When I visited Mark on Saturday morning, October 7th, I had to shower him because he and his bed were soaked with urine. After I had adjusted the water temperature, the water suddenly became very hot. If I had not had my hand in the stream, it could have been very dangerous for Mark. After many more attempts to regulate the temperature without success, I had to shower Mark with cool water. I mentioned this to the CNA, and he said that he was aware of the difficulty in adjusting the shower water temperature. I notified the AA that the problem needed to be addressed.

On October 9th, the administrator informed me that he had purchased a shaver for Mark and would keep it in his office overnight to charge it. The same day a new shaver was bought, the social worker informed me that Mark's shaver was found in the room across the hall from his room. The social worker placed it in a locked drawer that was provided for Mark. The key for the drawer was to be stored in the office.

Wednesday, October 18th, I sent the following email to the AA and copied the social worker and the DON.

Today when I visited Mark at 10:40 a.m., he was lying in bed in his gown. He was soaked with urine; his teeth were not brushed, and he had had no personal hygiene care. His breakfast tray was still sitting on the bedside table, even though the food had been eaten. Mark's partial denture was in his mouth, evidence that the evening shift had not removed it the night before and had not provided his evening dental care.

Mark's wheelchair was not in his room, so he could not go to the bathroom. I shaved Mark while he was in bed, then three aides came into the room (#1, #2, and #3). They found Mark's wheelchair, and #3 was going to take Mark to the shower. #1 attempted to get Mark out of bed. She kept telling Mark to "bend your leg," although Mark has a plate and screws in his leg, and it is practically immobile. I informed the caretakers of Mark's unbendable leg and showed the proper way to have Mark transfer to his chair.

After #1 removed the urine-soaked bedding, she proceeded to make the bed with clean linens without cleaning the urine from the mattress. After she had made the bed, I asked her if she had wiped down the mattress, and she said she had not. I told her that putting the sheets on a dirty mattress contributed to the bad smell in the room. She removed the bedding, cleaned the mattress, and re-made the bed.

When he took Mark to the shower, I asked #3 if he was aware of how the water temperature fluctuated in the shower. He said that he was and always had to adjust the water temperature. #2 told me that she had worked at Elm Fork for nearly four years, and the showers had always been like that. Can you imagine how much time would be saved if the water temperature did not have to continually be adjusted while showering the residents?

The paper towels are still lying on the toilet tank. They continue to fall out of the holder. This problem was mentioned in a previous email.

Note: The requests in the attached messages have not been addressed.

Suggestion: Make the staff aware of each resident's needs and be sure the staff receives the proper training to address those needs.

Thanks for your help…CN, MO's Mother

The previous requests were regarding Mark's dental care, his bathroom prompts, the shower water temperature, paper towel issue, a broken soap dispenser, the feces I had found on Mark (his hands, wheelchair, in his pants, and on his clothing), and Mark being unshaven. If these inadequacies seem minor to you, consider that they are ongoing and fail to be resolved.

Conditions remained unresolved throughout November.

December 1, 2006, it was announced that Elm Fork was under new management and had a new name: Carrollton Health & Rehabilitation Center (CHRC). That same day, I found the following when I visited Mark:

1) His partial denture was on the floor.
2) He was not wearing his eyeglasses.
3) His electric toothbrush had not been used.
4) He was eating lunch with his jacket on.
5) He was unshaven.
6) He was wearing taped diapers instead of pull-ups.
7) His hairbrush was missing.
8) There were no paper towels in the bathroom holder.

Mark had lost approximately 14 pounds since he arrived less than three months earlier. I continued to find fortified pudding snacks on Mark's tray table that had not been eaten. I reported these issues to the DON, and they were addressed at Mark's Care Plan Meeting on December 20, 2006. All but the dental care issues were resolved.

January 23, 2007, his doctor requested that psychological services be made available for Mark through Deer Oaks Behavioral Health Organization.

When I arrived at CHRC the next day, Mark's nurse and I made several observations.

1) Mark was lying in bed with the bed rails up. Mark was capable of transferring himself, and this prevented him from getting out of bed.

2) He was wearing no clothing from his waist down. (I understood this was the policy for bedridden patients. However, Mark had been at CHRC for over four months, and the staff should have been aware that this policy did not apply to him.)

3) The second finger of Mark's right hand had a **CIGARETTE BURN** that was not healing and appeared to be continually burned due to exposure to the ashes of his cigarettes. (The human resources director made a note for a cigarette holder to be purchased for Mark; this would allow his hand to heal, as it would not be continuously exposed to the live cigarette ashes.)

4) He was unshaven. By three o'clock in the afternoon, it seems that all routine personal hygiene tasks should have been completed. Mark's caretakers had been instructed to monitor Mark as he shaved with his electric shaver, which was stored in his bedside chest's locked drawer.

5) Urine-soaked clothing was in his closet, which produced a nauseating stench. (The nurse took the bag of clothing to the laundry.)

6) There was a urinal sitting on Mark's computer table. Mark never used a urinal. A sign on his wall was to remind his caretakers that he use the bathroom every two hours and before each smoke break.

7) The batteries in his CD player were dead, even though the nurse on duty was responsible for replacing the batteries each day.

I helped Mark dress, and we went to the smoking area for the 3 o'clock smoke break. The smoking monitor told me that Mark had no cigarettes. Instead of in the container where they were usually kept, four packs and a partial were found in the cigarette storage area.

On January 27th, Mark's diet was upgraded to Mechanical Soft, and his liquids were nectar-thickened. He would have a barium swallow exam in a week to ensure the diet was safe for him.

When I arrived at CHRC at 1:00 p.m. on February 1st, Mark was on his way to his room and was soaked with urine. In his room, the stench of urine was overwhelming. His CNA informed me that the smell was coming from Mark's roommate. I reported the smell to the DON, and she promised to have someone clean up the roommate. The batteries were dead in Mark's CD player, and someone had removed the batteries from his clock on the wall. There were spilled liquids on his computer desk. (The caretakers disregarded the huge sign on the wall above his desk that says, "Do NOT put liquids on this table!") I promptly emailed the administrator and social worker my findings.

Despite the inadequate care that Mark received, he continued to progress. Computer equipment upgrades kept his mind alert, and his fine motor skills were improving. He attended groups sponsored by Deer Oaks, which alleviated his anxiety. He gained several pounds and maintained a stable weight. His handwriting was legible, and by August 2007, he wrote short letters to his Grandma Brown. I picked him up every weekend, so he could spend either Saturday or Sunday at our home.

On the 28th, after he fell in his bathroom, Mark was admitted to the Medical Center of Plano, where it was discovered that his left leg had a hairline fracture. Instead of a hard cast, he was to wear a "soft splint" and bear no weight on his leg for three weeks. Two weeks later, I found Mark without the splint on his leg.

Regardless of my frustrations with the decline in Mark's daily care, we were able to contend with the inadequacies until, that is, the unsafe situations became too dangerous to disregard. Throughout the remainder of 2007 and into 2008, conditions deteriorated. Hot water in Mark's bathroom sink was unable to be regulated. The brakes no longer worked on his replacement wheelchair; a steep and slanting sidewalk that led to the smoking area made it necessary for someone to push Mark there. Over the next few months, Mark had tipped over in his wheelchair at least three times (even with a staff member pushing him) until the administrator made arrangements to have Mark escorted to the smoking area via the front door. Mark suffered serious skin breakdown on his bottom and on the back of his upper thighs caused by the vinyl seat in the old wheelchair he was using. After months of requesting a new chair, on June 29, 2007, Mark received a new wheelchair with a nylon fabric seat. The cover for the ceiling vent in Mark's bathroom fell to the floor. Although a grab bar was requested, Mark used the towel bar in the bathroom as a grab bar–until the nails pulled out from the wall. When Mark became continent and no longer wore diapers, all his new underwear went missing from his drawer. Since Mark had been released from physical therapy, his posture rapidly declined. A front tooth of Mark's partial denture had been broken off for months, and the social worker was unable to obtain a dental appointment for him.

Mark had a CT scan of his head on November 16th, after tipping over in his wheelchair. Fortunately, he was all right.

In mid-May of 2008, Mark was taken to Trinity Hospital by

ambulance, where he was admitted into the intensive care unit (ICU). His blood pressure was 66/49, and he had a severe bowel impaction that had nearly led to an obstruction. He was in the ICU until May 20th, when he was transferred to a hospital room. Seven days later, on May 27, 2008, he was discharged back to CHRC.

When Mark returned to CHRC, both pairs of his shoes were missing. To accommodate his specific needs, Mark's shoes had to be special-ordered, so I purchased a new pair; CHRC covered their cost.

The hospital doctor performed a colonoscopy on Mark on June 6, 2008. The prep for the colonoscopy was done so poorly that the X-rays showed stool remaining in the colon. The doctor told me that Mark was "getting better," even though the colonoscopy results were unreadable. Uncomfortable with the treatment and poor results Mark received from the doctor, I contacted my personal colon specialist (PCS). He had removed a cyst from Mark three years prior and was familiar with his medical history. On July 2, 2008, I notified Elm Fork and the hospital that Mark was changing doctors.

When I spoke with Mark's physician at CHRC, she was unaware of Mark's recent health issues, including his being in ICU, his extended hospital stay, and his elimination problems. It appeared that she had no communication with her physician's assistant (PA), who had apparently been writing orders without the doctor's knowledge. Needless to say, I immediately re-established his former doctor as Mark's physician.

Communication between weekday and weekend nursing staff was horrible. The weekend staff was unaware of the order for Mark to receive daily enemas until I asked the nurse. He discovered it when he looked through the records. My personal colon specialist (PCS) continued to follow Mark and successfully treated his colon problems.

On July 15, 2008, Mark was admitted to Plano Medical Center for his elimination problems. Unfortunately, when I removed his left stocking, I discovered that his ankle was red, swollen, and hot to the touch. He nearly went through the ceiling with pain when I touched his foot. In addition to the abdominal X-ray, I asked that they also look at his left ankle. Sure enough, his ankle was broken in three places. When I asked Mark if it hurt when his aide put on his shoe and sock that morning, he said, "Yes." I had noticed it was unusually difficult for Mark to transfer into my car. I had been with Mark on Sunday and Monday, and there were no signs of pain, redness, swelling, or heat in his left ankle. That indicated to me that his ankle had been broken between Monday afternoon and Tuesday morning. Apparently, Mark's caretaker did not recognize these obvious symptoms when she dressed him Tuesday morning. I asked the administrator to see if he could find out what happened. On July 16th, the administrator informed me that CHRC was in the process of doing an investigation.

The blatant disregard for patients' safety could no longer go unheeded. It would be too risky to allow Mark to return to CHRC. The hospital social worker found a nursing home where Mark would reside upon his discharge from the hospital.

CHAPTER 14

A Challenging Six Years
July 2008–March 2015

AFTER SPENDING 13 days in Plano Medical Center, on Monday, July 28, 2008, Mark was admitted to The Plaza at Richardson, Richardson, Texas (The Plaza). I looked forward to getting Mark settled into his new home. The Plaza was a non-smoking facility, which made me very happy. No more cigarette burns!

The meeting coordinator, director of social services, director of rehabilitation (physical therapy), the activity director, and a wellness specialist attended Mark's first Care Plan Meeting on August 14, 2008. The status of Mark's bowel problems, the sores on his bottom, and his broken ankle were not discussed. I was told these were nursing issues, and I needed to ask the nurse about them. That was unlike previous care plan meetings I had participated in where all topics of concern were addressed.

August 26, 2008, was my first email to the director of nursing (DON). Here are the four concerns I spoke to in my email:

1. When I arrived at 12:30 p.m., although we had discussed it the day before, Mark's urinal was overflowing, and his sheets and

gown were soaked with urine. (A sign had been placed on the wall to remind the staff to empty the urinal.)

2. Mark was confined to bed until his broken ankle healed; he was not to bear weight on his leg. Apparently, the CNAs were not informed of Mark's inability to get out of bed because, when I would arrive at The Plaza, Mark's morning drinks were sitting in a glass on the nightstand across the room. Someone needed to help him with his beverages.

3. Mark was to have milk on his food tray, but every day the CNA had to return to the dining room to get it.

4. Although I placed a denture tablet on top of Mark's denture cup, it remained there for several days, evidence that his denture had not been cleaned but stayed in his mouth over several nights.

I accepted that I would be facing the same failings of the staff over and over, as I had found in prior nursing homes. I wondered, "Was I enabling the staff every time I emptied Mark's urinal and changed his urine-soaked clothes and bedding? Did I prevent them from learning how to properly care for their residents?"

I noticed changes in Mark on August 28, 2008. He seemed confused, was very tense, and had difficulty turning in bed. He had hand tremors so severe that he could barely place his silverware in his mouth when he ate–usually side effects of over-medication. To avoid these side effects, Mark's blood level of his psychotropic meds needed to be monitored more frequently.

Although the orthopedic surgeon had put Mark on bedrest until his broken ankle healed, I learned that staff members got him out of bed to weigh him on September 2nd. The wheelchair in which he was transported did not have a leg rest to support Mark's broken ankle. The prior month a portable scales with a lift was used to weigh him in his bed. This time, the people who weighed Mark said they had no choice and were adamant that all weights needed to be completed on the first of the month. Both the DON and assistant director of nurses (ADON) told me that either the electric lift was out of order or the batteries were not charged. It seemed that, for Mark's safety, they could have waited one more day to weigh him. I reported the staff's use of poor judgment to the Administrator.

September 7, 2008, Mark was admitted to Richardson Regional Medical Center with seizures. After four days of testing and observation, he was discharged on September 11th with his seizures under control.

The following week, the surgeon upgraded Mark's status so that he was no longer on bed rest. He began receiving therapy, and I was impressed with his physical therapist and his speech therapist's proficiency. On the 25th, I commended Mark's therapists in an email to the Administrator. I also noted four oversights that I asked him to address.

1. Shortly after noon, Mark was still in bed with his gown on.
2. His urinal was in place; however, it was full of urine. It eventually spilled over, soaking the sheets and his gown.
3. His teeth had not been brushed, and there was evidence that his partial denture had not been removed the prior evening and placed in his denture cup. (There was a sign on the wall to remind the staff to remove Mark's denture every evening.)
4. Two hairbrushes (one bristle, one vent) were missing from Mark's drawer. I gave a copy of the email to the ADON, because she had effectively solved previous problems. The administrator replied to my email; he stated that he had talked with the DON and the ADON, and they assured him that they would address my concerns.

On October 18th, Mark was taken to Richardson Regional Medical Center with seizures. He was discharged on the 21st.

At Mark's November 6, 2008, care plan meeting, attendees disclosed that Mark's caretakers were too busy to follow through on his bowel and bladder training program. I asked if Mark was ever offered a urinal, as I would find Mark still in bed, soaked with urine, after 10 o'clock in the morning. No morning care had been provided, and his breakfast was fed to him in his room instead of the dining room. I continued to find urinals in the bathroom that had not been properly rinsed, and they reeked of urine. I was disappointed by the inferior care provided by The Plaza's staff.

X-rays of Mark's left leg, knee, and foot, taken in January 2009, showed severe osteoarthritic changes and severe osteopenia. For him to stay mobile, it was imperative that he receive physical therapy. Since Mark no longer qualified for PT or RT at The Plaza, his doctor prescribed PT at an offsite location. He began his therapy at Wellness Care Center (WCC) on January 26, 2009. WCC provided transportation to and from his therapy every Monday and Wednesday. I attended many of his sessions and was happy to see how much he enjoyed them. He developed a renewed interest in others and interacted considerably well with his therapists.

Over the years, it became clear to me that all of the nursing homes in which Mark lived had provided outrageously substandard care. I resigned myself to the fact I would have to deal with Mark's ongoing incompetent care, and I vowed that I would advocate for him in the best possible way. I continued to visit him nearly every day and developed a good rapport with his caretakers. I familiarized them with Mark's capabilities, so they could proficiently meet his needs.

Mark continued to expand his interests. His computer provided him contact with the outside world and allowed him to stay in touch with his friends and family via email. His best friend often sent him personal videos on flash drives to watch. He watched music videos on his computer and listened to his favorite music on his iPod Shuffle. He carried on conversations with his caretakers and therapists, and his speech improved considerably.

On March 19, 2009, I emailed the ADON informing her that March 23rd would be Mark's last day of his outpatient rehab services. The wellness therapist recommended that Mark receive restorative therapy. I was asked by The Plaza to hold an in-service training session for Mark's CNAs. On March 26th, we reviewed wheelchair transfers, toilet schedules, and cleanliness. Many of Mark's new CNAs were not aware that Mark was able to use the bathroom by himself, nor were they familiar with the operation and care of his electric toothbrush and shaver.

At Mark's Care Plan Meeting on May 7, 2009, I reported that Mark was very sleepy most of the time, so his Depakote and Dilantin were decreased. Mark was going to be discharged from the activity department for a lack of interest. Instead of dismissing him from the activity schedule, I asked the director to have the wellness specialist explore things that may interest Mark. I suggested they offer him projects that he would look forward to and help create for him a sense of accomplishment. Several months later, the activity department scheduled domino and checker games for Mark to participate in with a fellow resident.

Saturday night, July 25, 2009, Mark was taken to ER at Richardson Regional Medical Center with seizures and was returned to The Plaza Sunday. He developed a fever on Sunday evening, and by Monday, it was 100.8°. His doctor ordered a chest X-ray and a urinalysis. The urine was collected at approximately 1:00 p.m. on Monday, July 27th, and the nurse on duty called the lab to have them pick up the specimen. When I asked for the results of the urinalysis the next day, the nurse said she would get them to me when the lab faxed them to her. That evening, she called to tell me that Mark's urine specimen was still in the refrigerator at The Plaza. THE LAB HAD NEVER PICKED IT UP! I was appalled that such critical information could be overlooked, potentially putting residents at risk. Needless to say, I reported the incident to the administrator.

By August 2009, The Plaza had a new interim administrator–the fifth administrator since Mark was admitted in July of the previous year. Neglect and unsanitary conditions remained unchanged. Many times Mark would not be served beverages with his meals, his caretakers did not remind him to use the bathroom every two hours as I had requested, and his clothing was not changed when it was wet. Each time I would visit, he would be soaking wet, and his wheelchair literally stank even though the seat pad had been changed several times. Although staff was supposed to monitor him when he drank his daily beverage, it would remain on his tray table untouched.

Mark was no longer having physical or restorative therapy. Since the Physical Therapy Department was unfamiliar with restorative therapy guidelines, I researched it on my own and learned there was no limit of Medicare or Medicaid days for it. I thought Mark qualified for RT and continued to ask for it. Meanwhile, I assisted Mark as he walked with his walker. Without our daily walk in the hallway, Mark would have received no therapy at all.

Teeth continued to fall out of Mark's partial denture. Even though they were replaced each time they fell out, I coordinated with the dentist to provide Mark with an entirely new partial. When supplies were depleted from a resident's room, CNAs would retrieve them from another resident's room–promoting the spread of bacteria and disease. Non-flushable sanitary wipes were being flushed and clogging up toilets, and wastebaskets were left with liners piled in the bottom.

On September 2, 2009, Mark was prescribed medication by his urologist, and a follow-up appointment was scheduled September 30th to check its effectiveness. When I asked for the nurse's report to take to the doctor, it was learned that THE MEDICATION PRESCRIPTION HAD NOT BEEN FILLED AND, CONSEQUENTLY, THE MEDICATION HAD NOT BEEN GIVEN TO MARK. The appointment had to be canceled.

We were given notice on October 21, 2009, by the director of social services that Mark had to be discharged from The Plaza within 24 hours and that there were no other alternatives. Mark would be taken by ambulance to the ER at the Medical Center of McKinney. When I arrived at the hospital, the person who interviewed Mark asked me why he was there. Mark did not meet any of the criteria to be admitted into the hospital. She confided to me that when a nursing home wanted to get rid of a resident, they would send them to the ER, hoping they would be admitted into the hospital. Once the resident was admitted, the nursing home did not have to take them back; it was called "DUMPING," a violation of the law. I took Mark back to The Plaza. His discharge instructions referred to dementia and Alzheimer's disease—neither of which Mark had been diagnosed with. The next morning I sent the administrator an email stating that the actions taken the previous night were in violation of the law. "There are stringent criteria to admit a person into a hospital, and Mark met none of these." I asked him to let me know if he would like to meet with me. I received no response. The Plaza could not discharge Mark since it would have been a violation of the law.

December 9, 2009, Mark had a rectal fistulotomy at the Medical Center of Plano. After surgery I returned to The Plaza with Mark, only to discover that the nursing staff had been looking for him. Despite his surgery preparations the day before, they were apparently unaware that he'd gone to the Medical Center.

Following his surgery, Mark was to be on bed rest for 24 hours. When I arrived at The Plaza on December 10th, just before 8:00 a.m., Mark was in the dining room. I returned him to his room and placed him in bed on his side. I discussed Mark's follow-up care with the nurse and the ADON.

I went to my car to leave but had forgotten an envelope. When I returned to pick up my envelope, Mark's CNA was pushing Mark down the hall in his wheelchair! According to her, they were headed to the dining room. I explained to her that I had just returned him to his bed and asked her who told her to take him to the dining room, to which she replied, "Nobody." She then went and informed the ADON.

Once again, I returned Mark to his bed and told the nurse that she MUST INFORM HER STAFF OF MARK'S CARE! She promised that she would, but I was reluctant to leave, because none of Mark's caretakers seemed to be aware of his situation. I felt totally helpless when I returned to the nursing home only minutes after my discussions with the nurse and ADON and discovered that the very things we had discussed moments earlier had already failed. HOW CRUCIAL TO IMPRESS UPON THE STAFF THE IMPORTANCE OF COMMUNICATION! Another caretaker had already showered Mark, and when he discovered the sutures, strings, and drain coming from Mark's surgical wound, he had to ask the nurse about them.

When I visited Mark on December 13th, I had to clean his surgical wound, because there were feces on the sutures and drainage tubes. I emailed the DON and explained that I had placed two squirt bottles in the bathroom for Mark's wound to be cleaned after he used the toilet, with instructions to fill the bottles with warm water and squirt gently on the anus (from the front) and the wound (from the back) while Mark was on the toilet. I asked that the staff be very careful not to pull out the sutures, and after the wound was cleaned, the nurse should apply antibiotic ointment to the area to prevent infection. HOW I WISHED THE STAFF WOULD ASSUME THEIR OWN RESPONSIBILITIES!

In January 2010, I placed the following ad on a local high school web site.

Needed: a high school student to assist my son with basic computer tips (intranet-online access) and help with his speech for an hour or two a day, five days a week at $20.00/hour. The schedule

*is flexible. My son is in The Plaza at Richardson Nursing Home at
1301 Richardson Drive, Richardson, Texas 75080. Please contact
me for more information by responding to this email at _______,
or call me on my cell phone _______.*

An intelligent, personable student replied to the ad and began
working with Mark toward the end of the month. They met several
weekdays at 4:30 p.m. and various times on Saturday. Mark thoroughly enjoyed being tutored by her and looked forward to their lessons
together.

Mark's best friend, Roz, also visited him from Iowa in January.
They spent several days together, reminiscing about their college days.
Roz could always lift Mark's spirits and make him smile.

Throughout February 2010, the care that Mark received continued to be inferior. I kept the administrator apprised of the ongoing
mistakes made by his staff so he could intervene if necessary and try to
resolve the problems.

March 10, 2010, Mark had another fistulotomy at the Medical
Center of Plano and returned to The Plaza the same day. When he
returned, I stayed in very close communication with the staff to ensure
his recovery went well.

In April, I had begun emailing copies of recent requests, issues, and
complaints that I had sent to the administrator and staff members of
The Plaza, to the State Director of Consumer Rights and Services. I
enlisted the help of the Texas Department of Aging and Disability
Services (DADS) to help me appeal a 30-day discharge notice dated
April 8, 2010, that I received from the administrator of The Plaza. At the
administrator's request, I met with him and the Social Services Director
(SSD). He claimed not to have received my email, asking to start a family
council, even though it was in his inbox when he checked. The SSD had
questions about why I wanted to start a family council, and it was then
that the administrator told me that Mark would have to move out of the

facility because he had hit someone there.

The discharge notice stated that Mark had "developed a pattern of behavior that jeopardized the safety of others." The incidents referenced, though, were not abusive but were reactive, so there was *not* a developing pattern. The attempt to discharge Mark from The Plaza was based on an incident instigated by the medication nurse, who held Mark's wheelchair from behind, so he couldn't move. He reached back, inadvertently striking the med nurse on his arm. There was also the mention of an incident the previous year. The representative from DADS said that if Mark had been a danger to himself or others, he would have received one-on-one care after the first incident in October 2009. A behavioral program would have been implemented with the psychologist, and a care plan would have been put in place, directing the staff on how to interact with Mark. None of that happened. After a Senior Source ombudsman met with the administrator and me, *the discharge was deemed as inappropriate and without proper cause.* On April 14th, I received the following email from The Plaza administrator.

"I have some good news. We met with TDADS today, and they do not think a discharge is warranted in Mark's situation. However, we will need to meet with you and Mark and discuss a plan going forward. Please let me know when you will be available tomorrow to have a meeting with us." (Note: A meeting never materialized.)

On May 1st, Mark's brother Kevin, Kevin's daughters Danielle and Mariah, and Danielle's boyfriend spent several hours visiting Mark at The Plaza. It had been several years since they had seen each other and they had a great visit.

I continued to make observations and suggestions to improve Mark's day-to-day living. One of my biggest concerns was that, even though there was a high risk of bowel impaction among nursing home residents, the reports of residents' bowel movements were missing. Mark was inclined to have bowel problems, and lack of elimination would go unnoticed for days. It fell on me again to report Mark's abdominal distention to the DON; if I hadn't, the nursing staff would not have known to take action to treat him. To prevent future incidents, I asked the DON to put the bowel movement information back into the CNA reports.

I worked closely with Mark's restorative therapists, demonstrating how Mark could walk with his walker with minimum assistance and how he was learning to perform activities of daily living on his own (dental care, shaving).

Friday, August 27th, I had such an unpleasant encounter with The Plaza's new administrator that our ombudsman asked me to send him a synopsis of our meeting.

The ADON and I stopped by the administrator's office to see if he would be in the next day. He invited us in; the DON was already in his office. Nearly as soon as we entered, he verbally attacked me, accusing me of standing at the "round desk," flailing my arms and yelling at the staff. I was shocked when he said he had considered calling the police. He continued to badger me about yelling at the desk, and I told him that these issues needed to be resolved privately, in an office, behind closed doors. I reminded him that I had many conversations with both the current DON and the previous one, in their office.

He wanted to know why I "constantly feel the need to train my staff?" After all we'd been through, it seemed apparent to me, but I responded, letting him know that it was because of the high turnover of staff. "The new employees do not know Mark's needs, and they are not trained, so I tell them."

Administrator (ADR) accessed the Texas Department of Aging Nursing Home Criteria on his computer. Where, he asked, did it say that his staff had to take care of Mark's iPod for him? I explained that was not the issue. "Today, we are discussing the urine-soaked wheelchair, pants, bed, and floor."

He continued, asking, "What makes you think you can demand my staff take care of your son?" I explained, "I'm not demanding–I'm requesting. As my son's advocate, I need to make sure he gets the best care. My method has been to make an observation, make a suggestion, and point out the benefits."

ADR sarcastically referenced my business email signature several times, saying, "Oh yes, you are an Executive Administrative Something." I respectfully asked him to please stop those remarks.

When he asked, "If we are taking such poor care of your son, why is he still here?" I responded, "All of you know the high turnover of staff in nursing homes. When Mark came here, he came from another nursing home with a severe bowel impaction and his leg broken in two places. You know that with the high turnover, the care is always changing. The DON's predecessor is no longer here, the ADON's predecessor is no longer here–even your predecessor is no longer here. I'm also keeping Mark here for my convenience as well." I explained that I worked only four miles away, making it possible for me to visit Mark daily.

He also pointed out that I was rude to employees and offended them. I asked the ADON if I offended her, as well, and she weakly replied, "a little." I apologized to her and asked both her and the DON to let me know if my questions or suggestions were offensive.

ADR went on, claiming that when the ADON told me that she would take care of a problem, I didn't believe or trust that she would. I assured him that I did NOT say that and that I had never worked with the ADON.

It seemed evident to me that both the DON and the ADON had been put in a difficult position, unable to dispute anything their boss said. I decided that I would no longer make requests at the nurses' station; instead I would take them to the ADR, the DON, or the ADON. Although he had not treated me with respect, as I had always done in my own professional life, the meeting ended amicably on my part; we shook hands, and I shared that I was hopeful the situation could improve. Unfortunately, though, he was not open to another meeting.

I met with the Ombudsman a couple of days later, and we discussed the ADR's and my conversation.

In January 2011, I had another challenging exchange with ADR. At 2:00 p.m. January 21st, I went to The Plaza to pick up Mark for a doctor's appointment. Mark's roommate was upset, striking the air with his fists, and speaking to me in a different language. I didn't have time to try to understand why he was upset, so when I got to the doctor's office, I called his daughter and asked her if she could call her father and find out what was wrong. She told me that her father had moved to another room, so I thought his problems were resolved. As we were leaving the doctor's office, I noticed I had a voicemail on my phone. It was from the social services director at The Plaza. She told me that the Administrator (ADR) wanted to meet with Mark and me as soon as we got back to The Plaza. During the meeting, ADR told me that Mark had hit his roommate. Mark insisted that he had not. but ADR claimed that the roommate's sister and an interpreter had told him. Although no one observed any hitting, ADR stated that Mark would be discharged and that Mark needed me to serve as his "one-on-one." When I expressed that I had a job and worked every day, ADR said that he would appoint a staff member but that it would be unfair to the rest of the staff. A person from Timberlawn Hospital would come to The Plaza later that evening and evaluate Mark, then he would be taken by ambulance and admitted to Timberlawn. I asked that I be called when Mark was ready to leave, so I could follow the ambulance and be there to support Mark. At 6:00 p.m. I went home to wait for ADR's call.

At 8:10 p.m. I called ADR to find out the status of the evaluation, and he told me that the evaluator was currently interviewing Mark and was nearly finished. I drove to The Plaza, but when I arrived, ADR was gone. I introduced myself to the evaluator and asked her if Mark would be admitted; she indicated that she didn't know. Her license only allowed her to do an evaluation; a licensed psychiatrist would have to admit Mark. We talked about Mark's history; she told me that this hospitalization would be a voluntary commitment and that he didn't meet the criteria for OPC (Outpatient Psychiatric Care). After much back-and-forth and several phone calls, it was decided Mark would not be going to the hospital.

It was late when I left The Plaza. The evaluator was to call ADR with the results. Not long after I left, I received a call from the nurse at The Plaza telling me that ADR wanted to see me the first thing the next morning, which was a Saturday. I received yet another call, canceling; they would call me on Monday to reschedule.

My ombudsman joined me at the rescheduled meeting on February 11, 2011, that ADR had arranged. Nearly every member of the staff attended the meeting, including the janitor. At the meeting, ADR presented a letter for Mark and me to sign.

The letter stated that The Plaza was permitted to discharge Mark for the following reasons:

1) the transfer or discharge is necessary for Mr. Ostrander's welfare, and his needs cannot be met in the facility,
2) the safety of individuals in the facility is endangered, and/or
3) the health of other individuals in the facility would otherwise be endangered.

It continued: "We believe that Mr. Ostrander's behavior justifies discharge under this regulation; however, we have elected to forego discharge at this time, provided that you both indicate in writing that:

1. Mr. Ostrander will conduct himself appropriately in the future; and
2. he will complete the mental health assessment with Dr. ___; and

3. he will be compliant with any interventions or medications recommended by Dr. ___ or other of his treating physicians.

After deliberating with the Ombudsman, we opted not to sign the letter. And that was the end of that.

Mark spent from April 14 through April 26, 2011, in Methodist Richardson Medical Center for seizures and a severe lung infection, discovered when he was admitted. He was also dehydrated, and his electrolytes were out of balance. Additionally, he pulled out his Foley catheter (with the bulb inflated!) and did significant damage. That added several days to his hospitalization while he healed.

Mark went to Methodist Richardson Medical Center once more in 2011. On October 9th, he was taken to the emergency room for seizures but was able to return to The Plaza that same day.

Mark's next hospitalization at Methodist Richardson Medical Center on Thursday, April 5, 2012, was a nightmarish experience. Mark went to the emergency room for seizures. It took 5 attempts to intubate him, and during these attempts, staff used a contaminated bagging mask and suction tube. I later reported the unsanitary procedures to the Quality and Risk Manager, who followed up on the infection control issues in the Emergency Department. She sent me a certified letter stating that the Infection Control Practitioner re-educated both the Emergency Department and Cardiopulmonary Services staff on Infection Control practices.

From the ER, Mark was moved into ICU. I told the staff that Mark had a history of pulling out IV tubes and catheters. That night he extubated himself. Over the next seven days, Mark continued to pull out his nasogastric and IV tubing, including his Dobhoff NG tubes and PICC lines. They were repeatedly re-inserted when the doctor finally suggested that Mark have a sitter until the end of his hospital stay. He was discharged on April 17, 2012.

Mark was in MRMC on September 3rd, 4th, and 5th, for seizures, and again from October 16th through 19th, that time for fractured thoracic and lumbar vertebrae. Following his spinal fractures, he needed to receive physical therapy; however, his Medicare services were going to end on November 2nd. The rehab manager promised to give Mark all the therapy they were allowed to under Medicare. They would make sure he went on a Restorative Nursing Program and a Functional Maintenance Program. Physical Therapy lasted until December 18, 2012; Restorative Therapy picked Mark up from December 19th for one month, and Maintenance Therapy began January 20, 2013. Getting therapy for anyone on Medicare and Medicaid was extremely difficult. Mark's Rehab Manager worked closely with her staff and the Business Office Manager to make it happen. They were dedicated people!

Throughout 2013 Mark maintained his daily routines. Besides walking with his walker in the hall every day, he was memorizing songs on his guitar and playing his harmonica. He would take his guitar to a friend's room and play the melody of "Love Me Tender," by Elvis Presley, to him, while I sang the words. His friend could not walk or speak but would give a "thumbs up" to let Mark know that he enjoyed it.

On October 12th, he was diagnosed with pneumonia, dehydration, a urinary tract infection, and a rectal fistula. 2013 had been a tough year, but he managed to survive.

Cousin Joel from Minnesota, Martin, and I visited Mark Monday, December 30, 2013. Mark was delighted to see Joel and showed him his daily routine. Mark was in a good mood both the next day and Wednesday, New Year's Day, 2014, when Joel and I visited him. Thursday, when I saw Mark, he hadn't eaten, so I gave him some liquids. At about 5:00 p.m., Mark's nurse called me at home and said that Mark was agitated, wouldn't eat, wouldn't take his medicine, wouldn't go to his room, and was playing his harmonica loudly in the reception area. Joel and I went to The Plaza, and Joel convinced Mark to go to his room, lie down, and take his Vancomycin through his PICC line.

Friday, I visited Mark in the afternoon, and Joel visited later that evening. I requested that the doctor increase his psychiatric medication. Saturday, Mark wouldn't eat or take his medicine, so I went to The Plaza to help him with lunch. His nurse said that Mark had received a medication update, but that she didn't give it to him "because he didn't need it." BIG MISTAKE!

Sunday, January 5, 2014, I went to the Plaza at the social worker's request. Mark wouldn't eat or take his medication again. *Another attempt to discharge Mark was taking place.* We met with the administrator and ADON. Mark took his meds, but the administrator informed me that Mark would have to be discharged from The Plaza. He was picked up by ambulance at 11:20 a.m. and transported to Baylor Garland Emergency Room. Blood and urine samples were taken; Mark met with the social worker (SW), who contacted Timberlawn to give Mark a psychological evaluation. When the evaluator arrived at the hospital, she tried to get Mark admitted into a psychiatric unit for a few days to get his medication adjusted. None of the ten hospitals she called would take Mark because he had a PICC line. Mark had three days left on his prescribed Vancomycin, after which other facilities would be able to take Mark. During the ER visit, Mark did not create any problems, acted appropriately, and slept most of the time. An ambulance transported Mark back to The Plaza, and the ADON called to tell me that Mark had to be sent to Presbyterian ER because his drug test came back positive for cannabis (marijuana) and opiates. So, Mark was sent to Presbyterian ER via ambulance for a second drug test. I did not accompany Mark this time, but called and spoke with Mark's nurse, who agreed to call me with results. At 1:00 a.m., he called to let me know that Mark had had a psychological evaluation (even though that's not the reason he went there) and that he didn't meet the criteria to be hospitalized. He also told me they did not test Mark's urine for drugs, because The Plaza was able to do it.

The next morning, Monday, January 6th, I arrived at The Plaza between 10:30 and 11:00 a.m. Mark had eaten breakfast, taken his meds, was stable, and not creating any disturbance; a CNA was assigned to stay with him at all times. Mark ate lunch while I met with the administrator and ADON. I requested a second urine drug test to confirm the accuracy of the first. The administrator ignored the request and noted that Mark had to be discharged that day. I was given a letter that inferred that Mark could be discharged to a shelter or emergency room. In the meantime, the staff was calling other nursing homes to find a place for Mark, without success.

I had been in contact with the Assistant ER Director from Baylor Garland discussing a possible mistake regarding the urine test results. They continued to investigate. The Plaza's administrator suggested that the hospital re-test Mark's urine; however, after a patient was discharged, all samples were discarded. She contacted Mark's doctor and requested a new urine drug test. The administrator asked for her letter back from me to edit. Realizing it was invalid, she never brought it up again. Mark was not discharged. Instead, she told me they were going to do 15-minute checks on Mark, search his room daily, and not allow anything brought to him from outside The Plaza.

The next day, the nurse told me that since the requested urine analysis was not tested for drugs, it would have to be re-done. I asked Mark's status, and she said he was doing fine. I had contacted our ombudsman, and she told me that Mark could not be discharged to a shelter or emergency room. He would have to be released to a nursing home. She advised me to file a grievance complaint for use of tactics for improper discharge with the State of Texas, but I opted against it.

Mark's drug results came back positive. The ADON confirmed it was a *False Positive due to medicine that Mark was taking at the Plaza!*

Mark had been growing his hair for years and had the most beautiful long locks. His dedicated caretakers would braid his ponytail after every shower. He loved his long hair; it had become an integral part of him for which he received many compliments. In August 2014, he made the significant decision to donate his hair to be made into wigs for cancer survivors. He seemed sad the day he had his hair cut; he would be losing something that had been a part of him for so long. The organization representing the American Cancer Society sent Mark a letter of heartfelt appreciation for his generous contribution, which he proudly displayed on the wall of his room.

Mark was taken to the emergency room at the Medical Center of McKinney, TX, on the 6th of December with the intent to manage his psychotropic medication. He was not psychotic, but he had been depressed and expressed suicidal thoughts. He was admitted into the hospital, where he was closely observed, and his medications were updated. He was discharged 9 days later.

There was one more hospitalization for Mark in 2014. On December 23rd, he had hit another resident, so was taken to Medical Center of McKinney, and then transferred to the Wysong Psychiatric Campus. Mark was cooperative and established a good rapport with the staff. He was allowed visitors twice during the week and on weekends. I asked if Mark would be allowed to return to The Plaza, and the Wysong staff advised me that the nursing home must give a 30-day notice if they planned to deny Mark's return; otherwise, it would be considered illegal "dumping." Mark didn't enjoy the mental hospital atmosphere of Wysong and was eager to return to The Plaza. He was discharged back to The Plaza on the last day of the year, December 31, 2014.

It was becoming more and more difficult to tolerate the deteriorating conditions at The Plaza. Mealtime issues abounded. Residents were being served the wrong diet. Those who needed help to eat were overlooked and not being fed. Residents who were unable to propel their wheelchairs were left to sit at the dining room tables long after they had eaten and their dishes had been removed. Dining Room volunteers were resented by staff members who were resistant to change, resulting in disorder, confusion, and inefficiency.

In the residents' rooms and in the hallways, clean-up of spills and broken glass were not dealt with promptly and created hazards for the residents, staff, and visitors. Family members were hesitant to complain for fear of retaliation against their loved one. The Plaza was losing residents.

I, too, was searching for another place for Mark to live. By March 20, 2015, I had moved Mark to The Hillcrest in Plano, Texas.

CHAPTER 15

The Hillcrest

March 2015–November 2016

THE STAFF AT The Hillcrest was very accommodating. Because Mark's computer was such an essential part of his life, he was given a room near the server so he could access the web.

Mark soon settled into a daily routine of walking down the hall with his walker while I accompanied him. He documented the distance he walked each day on a chart he and I created on his computer–always striving for an extra foot or two. He also recorded each time he took his medicine on a separate chart. He learned how to put formulas in the cells that would automatically total his medicine for the day. Mark loved playing the card game Solitaire on his computer. He became very proficient at it and won nearly every game. He kept in touch with his friends and relatives via email and watched music videos on his computer. I brought him movie CDs from the library that he thoroughly enjoyed watching.

Several times a week, Mark would telephone Roz, and, even though Mark's speech was compromised, I was there to interpret. These conversations were a highlight of Mark's day. Roz would recommend videos and movies for Mark to watch, and they would reminisce about their college days.

Mindy and Mark were communicating nearly every day via email. They conspired to write a song together, each of them contributing a line at a time. This inspired Mark to extend his walks in the hallway. When he reached the end of the hall, he would stop and recite the words to their song, "How Nice Life Could Be," while he stood leaning against the wall before he walked back to his room.

> *"Whenever you are on my mind,*
> *And you seem so near to me,*
> *I leave bad memories behind,*
> *And think how nice life could be."*

A highlight of Mark's day was to take his harmonica into the dining room and play before lunch or dinner. His music always brightened the atmosphere. His fellow residents encouraged Mark to play and showed their appreciation with a round of applause after his short "concerts." Mark lived for the applause. He made many friends and introduced me to the people he had met in the dining room.

The more Mark improved, the more he realized that he no longer wanted to live. I think he feared that he would never fulfill his goals of becoming a professional entertainer or getting married and having a family.

Many times, when I visited Mark, I would find him lying in bed. "Hi, Mark, What are you doing?" His response, "Committing suicide." If he didn't eat, drink, or take his medicine, he believed he would starve and eventually die. Without his meds, he would have seizures, which would put him in the hospital where, since the condition was reversible, he would be right back where he began. Often, we treated it humorously, "That might take a while," and we would end up laughing.

Mark became progressively more depressed and was easily frustrated. Monday, June 8, 2015, he was admitted to Oceans Behavioral

Hospital to treat his depression. I visited him every day during visiting hours. There was a big difference between the care he was given at Oceans and the care he had received at The Hillcrest. It was obvious the Oceans staff was not accustomed to treating patients with such extensive medical issues as Mark. Although I showed them how to transfer Mark from his wheelchair, the day after he was admitted, his left leg and foot were injured. I met with his doctor, who prescribed an antibiotic for cellulitis. She mentioned that Mark coughed a lot when he took his medicine. Mark was on a pureed diet with thickened liquids, and his medications needed to be crushed or liquid. I noted that Mark had not had his teeth brushed or had his partial denture placed in a denture cup at bedtime the previous night.

When I visited Mark on Wednesday, he told me he had been given a cigarette. I told the nurse, who denied he had smoked. "He just thought he smoked." A different staff member later told me that it was he who had given Mark the cigarette.

Two technicians showed me how they had given Mark walk therapy by having Mark stand at the handrail and take side steps. I noticed that Mark could not place his left foot on the floor, so we tried to have him walk with his walker. He couldn't put any weight on his left foot at all, so I had him sit down and I removed his shoe and sock. He complained of pain when I pressed on the bottom of his foot and was unable to raise his left leg from the hip. I asked that the doctor order an X-ray of Mark's left leg and left foot. Up to this time, Mark had been receiving restorative therapy at The Hillcrest every day, during which he walked, assisted, with his walker, between 65 and 75 feet.

Mark had not had his teeth brushed nor had his partial denture been removed since before he was admitted. His breath was foul. That evening I called his nurse and asked her about Mark's leg. She said Mark had no complaints. I asked her to follow up on thickening his liquid medications and Mark's dental care.

Thursday morning, June 11, 2015, I spoke on the phone with the

DON and we discussed the four concerns I had: thickened liquids, the cigarette incident, leg X-ray request, and dental hygiene. I also told the clinical director and the therapist, so they were aware of those issues. During my visit that afternoon, Mark had a seizure. His anti-seizure meds had not yet been delivered.

Friday afternoon, there were still no results for the levels of medicine in Mark's blood. I'm not sure the nurses were even familiar with blood levels done for anti-seizure medicine. Mark's leg was improved, but no staff members were available to help Mark stand or walk.

Mark's Depakote and Keppra anti-seizure meds finally arrived Saturday afternoon, the 13th. I had to remind the nurse to mix his liquid medication with a thickener. Mark was still unshaven. His technician said she would shave him, and she also assisted while Mark walked approximately 25 feet on his walker. The rest of our visit was pleasant. Residents and family members joined us at our table in the main area; Mark was congenial and took part in the conversation.

Sunday, June 14th, Mark was in a good mood. He walked only a few feet because of pain in his left leg. For therapy, he did weight-bearing, and stood with his back to the wall for 15-20 minutes. He received no physical therapy the remainder of the week. On the following Friday, the DON said that the staff had walked Mark, but both Mark and the technician said that wasn't true. The DON would not allow me to walk Mark during visiting hours because, according to her, it was "too much stimulation." I checked Mark's left foot; the bottom was bruised, and he was still complaining of pain near his ankle. Mark's therapist informed me that Mark's discharge date of June 15th had been extended for a week because his doctor detected suicidal tendencies while they were in group therapy.

On Monday, June 22, 2015, I left a voicemail for the administrator asking her to verify that Mark had been receiving physical therapy by walking on his walker and standing, and asked her to check the status of Mark's left leg. I also asked if Mark's walker had been approved for him to use. I received no response to my voicemail from the administrator. When I visited Mark at 4:00 p.m., he was in a good mood. He said he had no exercise, walking or weight-bearing. I checked the bottom of Mark's foot; bruising was less, and his ankle was still sore. On Tuesday, I learned that the DON wasn't even aware that Mark's walker was in the facility. And then on Wednesday, she told me that the doctor said it was unsafe for Mark to walk with his walker. I suspected there was not enough staff to help Mark, especially since he had walked previously with assistance. Mark was receiving no PT at all. Instead, Mark and I did stretching exercises while sitting. When I removed his left shoe, there was blood on his sock; a scab had come off his toe. During my visit on Thursday, his sock was moist from his seeping toe.

My friend had visited Mark with me several times, and on Friday, June 26th, her relatives also visited. Mark thoroughly enjoyed meeting them. They laughed and shared many interests.

By Saturday, Mark's left leg was seeping from a blister, and his toes were still covered with a Band-Aid. Mark's breath was foul; he had not had his teeth brushed nor his partial denture cleaned. His technician said she would help Mark with his dental care if she had time. The nurse also said that if they had enough staff, they would help Mark walk with his walker. Later, the technician said that the DON told her not to walk Mark. So, no walking. Neither person knew where Mark's walker was within the facility. Lack of exercise exacerbated Mark's existing constipation problem. Mark asked how many days remained until his discharge from the hospital. He was eager to return to his healthier lifestyle. Sunday, Mark was very talkative and looked forward to his discharge, which finally happened on Monday, the 29th.

July 1, 2015, Mark poured his heart out in an email to his confidante, Mindy, whom he loved very much. His letter leaped from topic to topic, and he expressed some disturbing and radical views that seemed unlike him. He emptied his dresser drawers July 3rd, and reorganized all his belongings. He began to give away some of his possessions.

On July 7th, I received a call from his nurse; Mark was yelling and screaming and had hit his CNA. I called Mark's psychiatrist and scheduled an appointment for him to evaluate Mark. The next day, he adjusted Mark's psychotropic medication to alleviate his agitation.

I was elected president of the Family Council in June of 2016; the woman who was elected secretary was phenomenal. She entered into the meeting minutes, in great detail, each and every problem that was discussed at the meetings. As president, I made it a point to meet all of the family members of the residents in The Hillcrest and created a roster of residents and their family members. I recorded the issues on a chart where each concern was marked "Resolved, Partially Resolved, or Unresolved." Clearly marked on the chart was the following four-step procedure to resolve the issues.

Step 1 - Inform the DON or ADON of the problem. If unresolved by the next meeting, it was moved to...

Step 2 - Inform Management. If still unresolved, it was moved to...

Step 3 - Inform the Corporate Office, and finally, if unresolved, it was moved to...

Step 4 - Inform the State.

Residents were identified by names and room numbers, so their issues could be easily addressed. The chart, along with the meeting minutes, were distributed to the family members, administrator, DON, and ADONs. Improvements became evident over the next few months as we worked closely with the staff. The Family Council Meetings were well-attended, and family members were eager to share their issues.

On August 21, 2016, I reported an overwhelming stench of urine in Mark's room to the nursing staff and the administrator. They all gave conflicting instructions to the CNAs for the proper handling of Mark's roommate's catheter. I would find the catheter bag and tubing (with urine in it) in a plastic bag hanging from the bathroom shower rail. Sometimes, the catheter bag was emptied into a basin that was not rinsed, cleaned, or disinfected and was left sitting on the shower chair with urine in it. The bag with the tubing was sometimes stored in the bathroom and sometimes in the roommate's bedside table drawer. I informed the corporate office, and instructions were given to the staff for resolving the problem. At one point, the DON approached me and told me they could not do what Corporate asked. She said, "What are we supposed to do, hold the bag open until it dries out?" Finally, on September 10, 2016, the problem was solved by training one person to clean, disinfect, and air dry the catheter bag and tubing, while using another container to catch the urine from his catheter; then to clean and disinfect the container, place it in a double plastic trash bag and tie it to the bathroom shower rail. It took nearly a month to solve what should not have been a problem in the first place!

Due to his outbursts, Mark eventually ended up in a double room where he was the only occupant.

On November 14, 2016, Mark had become suicidal again and was transferred to Oceans Behavioral Hospital. Due to his suicidal tendencies, he would not be allowed to return to The Hillcrest upon his discharge. This meant that I had to step down as Family Council President. Our secretary also had to step down due to her overwhelming schedule. Very few people attended the December meeting, and it was decided to wait until March to hold the next meeting.

CHAPTER 16

The End of an Incredible Journey

December 14, 2016–December 26, 2016

BY MID-DECEMBER, WE were still searching for a place for Mark to live. It never became easier. The only place that would accept Mark was Victoria Gardens (VG) in Frisco, Texas; he was transferred there on December 14, 2016.

Constipation continued to be an issue for Mark, and on December 20th, his nurse added Senekot (2) and Dulcolax (1) to his regimen of laxatives. By 4 o'clock, Mark was very uncomfortable. His breathing was labored, and he was unable to defecate. The doctor removed some feces manually, then the nurse inserted three suppositories, gave him two enemas, and tried again to remove the feces digitally with little success. Mark was prescribed Miralax 3x/day and the liquid Magnesium Citrate. Mark was bleeding from his rectum.

Mark tolerated his pain so well! Even though he was extremely uncomfortable, he attended speech and physical therapy daily. His therapists were excellent, and he performed admirably in both speech and physical therapy. He walked 6 feet on his walker the first day and increased the distance each day.

Many of the residents at VG were unable to communicate, so I found Mark a tablemate in the dining room with whom he could converse. The gentleman said he played the harmonica, so I thought he and Mark may have something in common. Mark took his harmonica to the dining room, hoping to re-create an atmosphere similar to the one at The Hillcrest. My heart sank when Mark told me that a member of the staff told him to "Give it a rest" when he began to play.

On December 21st, the nurse told me that Mark had bowel movements all night; he was not bleeding, and his stools were large and liquid. The morning nurse did not give Mark Miralax because he was having too many bowel movements. Later that day, the Miralax was resumed. Mark was still very constipated; his stomach was distended and hard. He had had no normal, substantial, or firm BMs since he was admitted on December 14, 2016. The next day, the nurse reported that Mark had no pain, and his stomach was not as distended as it had been previously. I visited Mark every day, and when the CNAs told me that Mark had a BM, I would observe that he only eliminated tiny bits of soft stool. Considering the amount of food he was eating, his bowel movements should have been much bulkier.

December 23rd, at 2:15 p.m., the nurse practitioner ordered an X-ray of Mark's abdomen. At 3:15 p.m., the nurse gave Mark magnesium citrate and followed that with a suppository and an enema. At 11:00 p.m., the X-ray results showed no blockage. His colon, though, was full of stool.

Christmas Day, 2016, Mark's sister Lynn and her husband, Mark Ross, accompanied me to visit Mark at Victoria Gardens (VG). It was their first visit to VG, and Mark was thrilled to see them. He opened the gifts they brought him, showed them his computer set-up, and gave them a tour of the facility. I'm so glad they had such a pleasant visit as it would be the last time they would be able to talk with Mark.

When I arrived at VG on December 26, 2016, Mark was not interested in eating lunch and was obviously in pain, which became progressively worse throughout the afternoon. When his pain increased, the doctor prescribed Lactulose. With nothing else they could do, Mark was given the option of going to the hospital. I knew that Mark was hurting badly when he chose to go to the hospital; he disliked being in hospitals and would otherwise avoid going at all costs.

Mark was transported by ambulance to Baylor Scott & White Medical Center - Centennial, in Frisco, Texas. He arrived at 6:00 p.m. When he was in the emergency room, the nurse asked me what Mark had been given for pain. She was surprised when I told her, "Nothing," and immediately asked Mark what he would like for pain. Without hesitation, he responded, "Morphine." The X-rays showed that Mark had a perforated bowel, and part of his small intestine had necrosed. When the surgeon arrived, he explained that they would do everything they could to save Mark. They would need to remove much of his intestine, and if he survived the surgery, it was almost certain that he would end up with a colostomy.

Mark had been through hell over the past 22 years, and I couldn't imagine him bearing more pain and suffering than he had already endured. Mark did not want to be kept alive by artificial means. Without the surgery, his organs would slowly fail as the infection continued to spread throughout his body. The alternative would be for Mark to receive a continual morphine drip to end his pain.

Martin notified Lynn and her husband, who came directly to the hospital. Although Mark had already been sedated to control his pain, we continued to talk with him to let him know we were there. Shortly after the decision was made to not have surgery, Mark was moved to a private room. Lynn, Mark, Martin, and I stayed with Mark while the nurses attempted to insert an IV into his arm for the morphine drip. At 11:52 p.m., Mark's heart stopped. He had survived only six hours after he arrived at the hospital.

Although Mark had wanted to die for many years, he persevered through tough times and managed to pop back up with each setback. Mercifully, his wish was granted, and I felt so very sad, even though I knew he was where he wanted to be. Mark was finally at peace.

Mark willed his body to science, so, when he passed away, he was taken to The University of Texas Southwestern Medical Center (UTSWMC), where he contributed to medical education. He was involved in a course for Orthopedic Research and Surgery studies, which helped train Orthopedic Surgeons.

Mark was cremated and buried in the Memorial Garden on UTSWMC campus:

"In memory of those who have so graciously helped further the advancement of medical science."

A memorial service was held for Mark at our Family Reunion in Minnesota in July 2017. Binders of his artwork, poetry, and music were displayed, and videos of his life's journey were shown.

Mindy sent this remembrance of Mark that Martin read at his memorial:

At first, Oty was my brother's charming and good looking friend. Four of Roz's sisters had crushes on him. ☺ How could we not love him when he got our brother to take dance classes while they were attending NIACC!?! No way would we miss that dance recital!

And then he became MY special friend. I was going through some very hard times, and Oty had been facing some struggles of his own. My brother asked him to come and talk to me, and he did. He drove across part of the state just to help me, and he knew exactly what to say. He won my heart that day, not because he was gorgeous in so many ways--or because he was a phenomenal dancer--but because his manic depression had changed him, and he had become a more caring person.

We had a great talk that day, and I was very sad when I learned he tried to commit suicide a few years later. However, my brother and I got to know Oty better while he was in the nursing home. He would open up to me in emails and share his love of music. I also got to know his family, Colleen and Martin in particular.

Colleen never let him get away with being lazy. She made sure he got up and walked; sent emails even if he would rather live in his songs; and told him if he wanted to marry me, he would have to get a job first. Smiles ☺

He informed me he wanted to be an entertainer. I said, oh, have you been practicing on your guitar? No, he said, but it would be his job so we could get married. That is how I came to be his fiancée, even though I told him I have been married once and never wanted to do that again. LOL ☺

He had his mom send his ring, which was so big I put it on a chain. We fought like all couples when he said he wanted it back, and I told him no way! LOL That ring is being passed on to his nephew Zach. I am so grateful Mark Ostrander was part of my life. I will always remember him fondly.

Mindy (Malinda) Rosdail Johnson

Mark's Memorial Cards:

Dear Mark,

Your talent for music and dance became apparent by age seven when you competed in – and won – many musical events and dance contests.

Popular in school, you lettered in track, wrestling, and football, and represented your class as Homecoming King.

Your academic abilities revealed themselves through good grades from the time you began school (Honor Roll) throughout college (Dean's List) and achieved your Associate Degree in Science.

From age 21, you fought your toughest battle - bipolar disorder - and had to withdraw from your junior year in college. However, you persevered and went on to graduate with your Computer Technology degree.

I will treasure the time we had together from the beginning to the last years of your life. It feels like everything good is missing since you left – there's an emptiness. I hope you're dancing in the sky. I hope the angels know what they have. I'll bet it's so nice up in heaven since you arrived.

I Love You and Miss You,
Mom

Late Monday afternoon, after the reunion, Marge, Joanie, Laurie, and I went for a boat ride with Joel. Soaring toward us above the trees was a very large bird. It passed us, then circled back and flew alongside the boat for several minutes. It was a beautiful eagle! We sensed this eagle was a sign from Mark letting us know that he was flying free and dancing in the sky…

"Catch ya later, Mark"